Nurses' Aids Series

MATHEMATICS IN N

Nurses' Aids Series

Anatomy and Physiology for Nurses
Ear, Nose and Throat Nursing
Geriatric Nursing
Mathematics in Nursing
Medical Nursing
Microbiology for Nurses
Multiple Choice Questions, Book 1
Multiple Choice Questions, Book 2
Multiple Choice Questions, Book 3
Obstetric and Gynaecological Nursing
Paediatric Nursing
Personal and Community Health
Pharmacology for Nurses
Practical Nursing
Practical Procedures for Nurses
Psychiatric Nursing
Psychology for Nurses
Sociology for Nurses
Surgical Nursing
Theatre Technique

Special Interest Texts

Accident and Emergency Nursing
Anaesthesia and Recovery Room Techniques
Cardiac Nursing
Gastroenterological Nursing
Neuromedical and Neurosurgical Nursing
Nutrition and Dietetics in Health and Disease
Ophthalmic Nursing
Orthopaedics for Nurses

NURSES' AIDS SERIES

Mathematics in Nursing

Sixth Edition

Pamela M. Jefferies, SRN, RSCN, RNT

Director of Nurse Education, Normanby College, King's College Hospital, London

BAILLIÈRE TINDALL
LONDON

Published by Baillière Tindall,
a division of Cassell Ltd,
1 St Anne's Road, Eastbourne BN21 3UN

First published as *Arithmetic in Nursing* 1956
Fourth edition 1972
Fifth edition published as *Mathematics in Nursing* 1978
Reprinted 1981
Sixth edition 1983

ISBN 0 7020 1011 1

Typeset by Scribe Design, Gillingham, Kent
Printed in Great Britain by Spottiswoode Ballantyne Ltd., Colchester and London

---

British Library Cataloguing in Publication Data

Jefferies, Pamela M.
Mathematics in nursing.—6th ed.—(Nurses' aids series)
1. Nursing—Mathematics
I. Title II. Series
510'.024613 RT68

ISBN 0-7020-1011-1

Contents

Preface

It is now twenty-seven years since the original publication of *Arithmetic in Nursing*. During the intervening period the necessity for nurses at all levels to be numerate has increased considerably. Moreover, the safety of patients is frequently dependent on the accuracy of the calculations which are made.

When the plans for revising the book were being formulated, consideration was given to removing the early chapters which relate to the basic concepts of numeracy. The aim of these has always been to refresh the memories of those who have not used figures for some considerable time. However, some investigations amongst student nurses who had recently left school revealed that revision of fundamental principles was a prerequisite to their application to nursing. Consequently, much of the information has been retained, albeit in a format which is different from that used previously.

The metric system is now used throughout the book, but the chapters explaining the use of this and the Système International d'Unités (S.I. units) have been retained for the benefit of those who are unfamiliar with the topic.

As always, the purpose of the book is to assist student and pupil nurses with their studies. It is hoped, however, that trained nurses might also find that it can be used as a reference text.

A new chapter has been included in this edition about the need for numeracy amongst nurses. In an age of increased technology and sophisticated medical treatment, all nurses must be able to utilize figures if they are to care for their patients in the most effective manner. An attempt has been made, therefore, to elicit the many aspects of the work which involve the use of numbers. In the remainder of the text each topic has been related to its importance in the care of patients in order to emphasize to readers that without these skills they will be unable to ensure the welfare of those for whom they have to care.

December 1982 PAMELA M. JEFFERIES

1 The Need for Numeracy

The purpose of this book is, and always has been, to assist nurses to interpret and manage the figures they encounter. There is a common misconception amongst many people, that familiarity with figures is not an essential prerequisite for a career in nursing. It is true, however, that on entry to training, many students and pupils are dismayed when they discover that without this ability they are unable to fulfil their responsibilities efficiently.

Nursing is frequently considered to be an art. It is, however, much more than that. The technological age in which we live has caused the introduction into hospitals of very sophisticated equipment. So that this can be utilized effectively, the staff have to use figures and interpret their meanings.

In this chapter an attempt will be made to describe some aspects of nursing in which the use of figures is essential. It is hoped that this will demonstrate the need for the modern nurse to acquire the necessary skills so that she or he can care for her patients adequately. In addition, it should become evident that the need increases with advancement in one's career.

Drug administration

Everyone is aware of the fact that the administration of drugs constitutes a very large portion of modern medical treatment. There can be very few people who have never used drugs, even if it was only two aspirin tablets or a few vitamin tablets.

Many prescribed drugs are very potent. Moreover the nurse has often to calculate the required dose from a supply which is dispensed in a standard strength. This applies particularly in the care of sick children. If the nurse is unable to make accurate calculations, she or he is liable to give an incorrect dose to the patient. This could result in considerable harm to the person concerned.

Fluid balance

Many hospital patients require constant monitoring of their fluid intake and output. The responsibility for this falls on the nurse; and the doctor relies on the accuracy of the records so that he or she may prescribe the correct treatment. An error on the part of the nurse can therefore result in serious consequences for the patient.

Infant feeding

The responsibility for calculating the nutritional requirements of sick infants is frequently that of the nurse. Moreover, it is the nurse who has to explain feeding regimens to parents. Unless the teaching is clear and accurate, mothers will be unable to give the correct feeds to their babies. The result of this could be underfeeding, or the inclusion in the feeds of an excess of certain nutritional elements which might prove dangerous to the infants concerned.

In addition to the examples given above, the nurse has constantly to read and interpret figures.

Laboratory reports

The majority of laboratory reports are expressed in figures. It is necessary for the nurse to possess the ability to interpret these in order to care for patients adequately. Nowadays, the metric system and S.I. Units are the means whereby the results of many investigations are expressed. These topics will be discussed in later chapters, but it is imperative that individual nurses are familiar with them.

For laboratory reports to be used effectively it is essential that the reader is familiar with the normal variations in biochemical levels, so that those which are abnormal are quickly and easily discerned. Moreover, the nurse who is not aware that the figure 10^6 means 1 million, does not have the knowledge of very basic information. Without this, the complications of her work will be compounded.

Ward management

Increasing seniority brings with it the need for greater skill in the use of figures. To some people it appears that the reasons for this have little connection with the nursing care of patients. However, the ward sister who is unable to make simple arithmetical calculations discovers that her duty rotas are inaccurate. This may mean that staffing levels become imbalanced. This affects patient care directly. Another responsibility of the ward sister is to calculate bed occupancy figures. This also requires the ability to use numbers.

Middle management

Those nurses who are promoted to positions more senior than that of ward sister frequently complain that one of their major problems is that of estimating staffing levels. This difficulty may be due to the fact that there is a basic lack of familiarity with fractions and decimals, and an inability to multiply and divide. An example of this is the translation of hours worked by part-time staff into the number of whole-time staff that these represent.

For example, the calculation of the number of whole-time equivalents represented by 20 part-time staff can be estimated as follows:

10 part-time staff each work 20 hours each week
(This equals 200 hours)
10 part-time staff each work $17\frac{1}{2}$ hours each week
(This equals 175 hours)

$$200 + 175 = 375$$

If the working week for a full-time employee is $37\frac{1}{2}$ hours, it would require 10 full-time staff to give 375 hours work. Therefore, those 20 part-time staff are equal to 10 whole-time equivalents. From these calculations it is possible to estimate the cost of employing these people.

The above calculation required only the ability to multiply and divide, but without that skill, nurse managers are liable to experience considerable difficulties.

Senior management

Those nurses who progress to posts in senior management positions find that there is an increasing need to be numerate. This can be demonstrated by the fact that there are designated posts for nurses who are required to spend the majority of their professional lives working with figures, in order to determine such important issues as the numbers of staff required to care for patients, and the cost of this to the country.

In an age of economic constraints, budgeting features largely in the work of senior managers. The person who has the ability to interpret figures accurately and to understand statistics is at a considerable advantage.

It should be remembered that hospitals are financed from public funds and that the most effective and economical use of these is essential.

Nursing education

The nurse who decides to embark upon a career in nursing education will quickly find that in this branch of the profession numeracy is also required. The subjects studied as part of the training for teaching demand familiarity with figures. Moreover, tutors have to convey information to others. Unless they have good comprehension themselves it is not possible for them to transmit the facts to their students.

Senior tutors are required to use figures in a manner similar to their service colleagues, and without the ability to do so they are unable to function with full effectiveness. It should also be remembered that the allocation officer, who holds the responsibility for ensuring that nurses in training obtain the correct clinical experience, could not fulfil her or his duties without the ability to work with figures.

Research

During recent years the philosophy of nursing as a research-based profession has been advocated with increasing frequency. Many nurses now hold degrees, and are devoting their energies to research. This requires the ability to collate numerical information and to interpret it, which means developing skills in using statistical formulae. For those who read research reports, there is a need to understand the figures which are contained therein. Once again numeracy is required.

In the foregoing paragraphs an attempt has been made to indicate the need for numeracy amongst nurses. The following chapters will attempt to clarify some of the more important aspects of this; and to assist nurses in becoming familiar with figures and their uses. It is hoped that this will help them to give more efficient care to their patients.

2 Numbers, Prime Numbers and Factors

NUMBERS

For convenience the human race attaches labels to all things. That in itself makes communication possible. For example, when a person says 'book' everyone has some idea what he means. People in different occupations are likely to conjure up mental images of very different types of book, so we qualify 'book' with adjectives to restrict its meaning, e.g. a textbook. Thus a clear meaning is conveyed. Such convention is satisfactory until we wish to speak of cost and quantity. Then special adjectives, the numbers, are employed. These are as fundamental to our civilization as speech. Without them any sort of progress in commercial, scientific or social matters would be impossible.

A nurse uses numbers throughout the day. Bed states, estimating the need for and ordering of supplies, giving medicines and keeping charts of various types all require the nurse to be proficient in the use of numbers. Provided the rules are clearly understood and followed the manipulation of numbers is not difficult. The risk of error is reduced if the objects to which numbers refer are always borne in mind when making calculations.

The rules for dealing with problems consisting solely of addition and subtraction or division and multiplication will be familiar to men and women entering the nursing profession, but it would be wise at this stage to revise the procedure for handling mixed calculations. Sums consisting only of addition and subtraction can be performed in any order without the final result being altered.

Example

$$24 - 12 + 3 - 2 + 9 - 6 = 12 + 1 + 3 = 16$$
$$24 + 3 + 9 - 12 - 2 - 6 = 36 - 20 = 16$$

However, if the calculation involves multiplication or division as well as addition and subtraction, the order of work is very important if the correct result is to be obtained. The rule is to deal firstly with multiplication and division, secondly with addition and subtraction. There is an exception to this rule. Brackets are often used in calculations and those parts of the sum within brackets must be worked first. Sometimes it helps to put brackets around parts of the sum when dealing with multiplication and division.

Example
Consider the following expression

$$6 \times 12 + 216 \div 3$$

Using brackets this equals

$$\begin{aligned}(6 \times 12) + (216 \div 3)\\ = 72 + 72\\ = 144\end{aligned}$$

If the calculation had been performed in the order in which it was written there would have been an error of 48; a considerable difference. Brackets need not necessarily be inserted in this way once observance of the rule about the precedence of signs becomes a habit.

When removing brackets in calculations involving addition and subtraction the rule of signs must be remembered, viz. if the sum within brackets is preceded by a positive sign the signs within the brackets remain unchanged. If a negative sign precedes the bracket, the signs within the bracket must be reversed when the brackets are removed.

Example
Resolve the following expression

$$42 + 7 - (16 - 3) + 7 - (2 - 1)$$

The sums within the brackets can be worked first

$$\begin{aligned} &42 + 7 - 13 + 7 - 1 \\ &= 56 - 14 \\ &= 42 \end{aligned}$$

Alternatively the brackets can be removed

$$\begin{aligned} &42 + 7 - 16 + 3 + 7 - 2 + 1 \\ &= 60 - 18 \\ &= 42 \end{aligned}$$

In the above example, all the positive numbers were added together, then all the negative numbers added and the latter subtracted from the former.

Before leaving the subject of brackets we should remember that two sets of brackets side by side mean that the product of the first set is multiplied by the product of the second set, thus:

$$(2 + 4)(9 - 3) = (6)(6) = 36$$

From the rule of signs we can see that the product of two positive numbers or two negative numbers is a positive number, and that the product of a positive and a negative number is a negative number.

Example

$$(-6)(+6) = -36$$
$$(-6)(-6) = +36$$

Exercises

Now try these:

1. Of 240 patients 120 are visited at the week-end, 80 are visited mid-week, but 40 of these patients are visited at the week-end and mid-week. How many patients received no visitors?

2. $4 + 7 - (7 - 6) + 3 + (4 - 1) = \quad ?$

3. $7 \times 3 + 27 \div 9 - 3 = \quad ?$

4. $18 + 27 \times (12 - 9) - 90 = \quad ?$

5. $(7 + 6)(6 - 3) = \quad ?$

6. $(-6)(5 - 8) = \quad ?$

7. $90 \div (3 \times 5) = \quad ?$

FACTORS AND PRIME NUMBERS

Some numbers are seen to be the product of other, smaller numbers. For instance 4 is the product of 2×2, 8 is the product of $2 \times 2 \times 2$, six is the product of 2×3 and so on. These smaller numbers are called *factors* of the larger number. Obviously, any number has factors consisting of itself and 1, e.g. $17 = 17 \times 1$; $23 = 23 \times 1$, etc., but 1 does not really count as a factor. Numbers that have only themselves and 1 as factors are called *prime numbers* and it is important to be able to recognize them at sight. The smaller ones are easily recognized. They are 2, 3, 5, 7, 11, 13, 17 and 19. To recognize them when searching for the factors of a number saves a great deal of fruitless search.

Factors which are prime numbers are called *prime factors* and in many calculations it is essential that these are discovered in order that the solution may be found.

Example

10 is the product of 2 and 5, both of which are prime numbers;

42 is the product of 6 and 7;

7 is a prime number; but
6 is the product of two more, 2 and 3.
The prime factors of 420 are therefore 2, 5, 2, 3 and 7.
Arranging these in order we can say that

$$420 = 2 \times 2 \times 3 \times 5 \times 7$$

No amount of dividing will reduce these primes to any other factors.

The prime numbers up to 19 have already been stated above. There are many more; indeed, some mathematicians have spent years extending the list. Their work involves attempting to divide a number by all the known primes, and this involves long division as there is no short method. As far as nurses are concerned, only the smaller prime numbers are likely to be of use. It will be noticed that 1 is not included in the list of prime numbers. Unity is in a special category all its own. Further it will be noticed that 2 is the only even number in the list. A moment's thought will reveal why this is so. All other even numbers are divisible by 2. In other words, 2 is a factor of all even numbers; hence they cannot be primes.

Finding the factors of a number involves dividing the number by successive primes starting with 2. To make this task easier there are tests to which the number can be subjected. These are called the 'tests of divisibility'.

Division by 2. All even numbers are divisible by 2, so it can be stated that if the *last* integer of a number is divisible by 2, so is the whole number.

Division by 3. If the sum of the individual integers is divisible by 3, so is the whole number. For example, to discover if the number 241 842 is divisible by 3: Add the individual integers—$2 + 4 + 1 + 8 + 4 + 2 = 21$. As 21 is divisible by 3, so is the larger number. $241\,842 \div 3 = 80\,614$.

Division by 4. If the *last two* integers in a number are divisible by 4, so is the whole number.

Division by 5. Only numbers ending in 0 and 5 are divisible by 5.

Division by 6. All *even* numbers are divisible by 6 if the sum of their integers is divisible by 3. This test is compounded from the test for 2 and for 3, which are the factors of 6.

Division by 7. There is no test for 7 and the only way to determine if it is divisible is to divide by 7 in full.

Division by 8. If the *last three* integers in a number are divisible by 8, so is the whole number.

Division by 9. If the sum of the integers is divisible by 9 so is the whole number. This is similar to the test for 3.

Division by 10. Only numbers ending in 0 are divisible by 10.

Division by 11. This is rather an unusual test. The *alternate* integers are added together. The remaining integers are then added together. This of course results in two numbers. If they are equal, of if their difference is 11, the whole number is divisible by 11.

For example, test to see if 13 937 is divisible by 11:

Add alternate integers	$1 + 9 + 7 = 17$
Add remaining integers	$3 + 3 = 6$
The difference between these is	$17 - 6 = 11$

Therefore the number *is* divisible by 11:

$$11\overline{)13\,937}\quad 1\,267$$

Again: Is 897 437 211 divisible by 11?

$$9 + 4 + 7 + 1 = 21$$
$$8 + 7 + 3 + 2 + 1 = 21$$

The additions are equal, therefore the number *is* divisible by 11:

$$11\overline{)897\,437\,211}\quad = 81\,585\,201$$

These tests are applied to a number to determine its factors. Each test is applied in turn until the number is shown to be divisible by one of the primes. The number is then divided by this prime number and the resulting figure is tested again until another prime is discovered to divide. The division is carried out and the new figure is again tested. This is repeated until the last figure is itself a prime number. The prime numbers are then lined up and these are the prime factors of the number.

Examples
What are the factors of 112? (112 is an even number, therefore 2 is a factor)

$112 = 2 \times 56$	(56 is even, so 2 occurs again as a factor)
$56 = 2 \times 28$	(28 is even, so 2 occurs yet again as a factor)
$28 = 2 \times 14$	(14 is even, so 2 is a factor yet again)
$14 = 2 \times 7$	(7 is a prime number, so factors are now complete)

$$\therefore\ 112 = 2 \times 2 \times 2 \times 2 \times 7$$

What are the prime factors of 150? (150 is even, therefore 2 is a factor)

$150 = 2 \times 75$	(75 is odd, therefore 2 does not occur again as a factor. Test for 3: $7 + 5 = 12$. 12 is divisible by 3 so 75 must be)
$75 = 3 \times 25$	(25 is the product of 5 and 5, both of which are prime factors)

$25 = 5 \times 5$

$$\therefore 150 = 2 \times 3 \times 5 \times 5$$

Find the factors of 5775. (An odd number therefore 2 is not a factor. Test for 3: $5 + 7 + 7 + 5 = 24$, which is divisible by 3.)

$5775 = 3 \times 1925$	(1925. $1 + 9 + 2 + 5 = 17$. Not divisible by 3. Test for 5. The number ends in 5, so is divisible by 5)
$1925 = 5 \times 385$	(and again)
$385 = 5 \times 77$	(77 is the product of 7 and 11, both of which are primes, so the search ends)

$$\therefore 5775 = 3 \times 5 \times 5 \times 7 \times 11$$

Are the following numbers divisible by 11?

(1) 8 969 994 (2) 35 728

(*a*) Sum of alternate digits $= 8 + 6 + 9 + 4 = 27$
Sum of remaining digits $= 9 + 9 + 9 = 27$

$\therefore$ the number is divisible by 11.

(*b*)

$$3 + 7 + 8 = 18$$
$$5 + 2 = 7$$
$$18 - 7 = 11$$

$\therefore$ the number is divisible by 11.

Exercises

1. Which of the following numbers are primes?
(*a*) 6 (*b*) 7 (*c*) 4 (*d*) 3 (*e*) 9 (*f*) 13

2. Which of the following numbers are divisible by 3?
(*a*) 14 (*b*) 27 (*c*) 195 (*d*) 296 (*e*) 4311
(*f*) 178 465

3. Which of the following numbers are divisible by 11?
(*a*) 374 (*b*) 3740 (*c*) 9244 (*d*) 42 966
(*e*) 345 743 782
4. What are the prime factors of the following numbers?
(*a*) 12 (*b*) 14 (*c*) 35 (*d*) 38 (*e*) 138 (*f*) 380 (*g*) 924 (*h*) 525

3 Fractions

The numbers discussed so far are called natural numbers when referring to specific quantities of whole objects, and integers when negative and positive signs are attached. To enable us to deal with quantities less than whole numbers a special set of numbers called vulgar fractions was evolved. These, together with integers, are known as the rational numbers.

We mostly take for granted the use of terms such as 'a quarter of a loaf', 'half an hour', or 'three-quarters of a pint'. Such measurements are used frequently without us stopping to think that we are using fractions, things that are part of a whole and which tell us what we want to know in a concise and simple way. In hospitals we must be particularly careful to ensure that information is conveyed in a precise and exact manner. A vivid imagination is not needed to realize the unhelpfulness of giving a consultant vague information such as 'this patient has had a bit of morphia' or 'this patient has had deep X-ray treatment for part of an hour'.

Fractions such as one-quarter, one-half, three-quarters, and their numerical expressions $\frac{1}{4}$, $\frac{1}{2}$, $\frac{3}{4}$, are so familiar to one and all that detailed explanation is not needed. We use them in our everyday life when we talk of such things as quarter of an hour, half a pint, or three-quarters of a pound. Indeed, so familiar are they in such a context that the fact that they *are* fractions tends to be forgotten. On such homely examples can be built many of the fundamental facts that have to be mastered before the mystery is taken out of the manipulation of fractions.

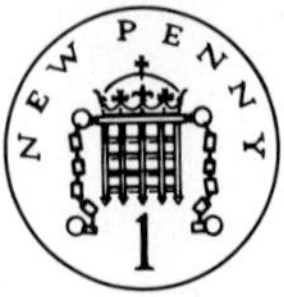

1 new penny

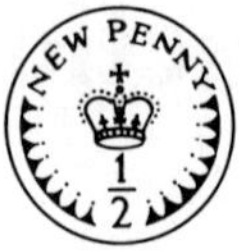

½ new penny

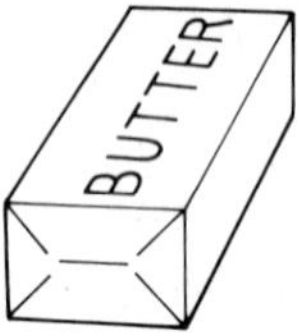

1 pound

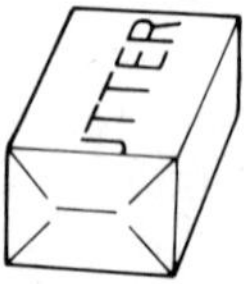

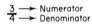

¾ pound

$\frac{3}{4}$ 3 ⟶ Numerator
4 ⟶ Denominator

4 parts, therefore
denominator is 4

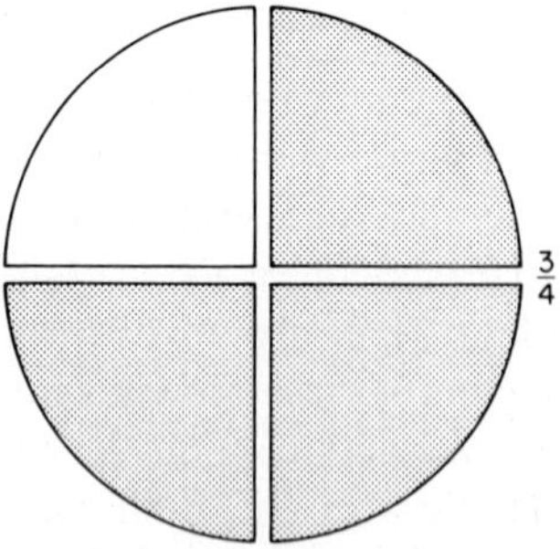

3 shaded parts, therefore
numerator is 3

Let us examine a fraction, any fraction, and see how it is built up and what information it gives us. $\frac{3}{4}$ consists of two numbers, set down one over the other with a line between. Three over four. The number under the line is called the *denominator* and tells us the number of parts in the thing that we happen to be dealing with. The denominator of any fraction will always give us that much information, whether it is small as in $\frac{1}{3}$, $\frac{1}{5}$, etc., or whether it is large as in $\frac{1}{1000}$, $\frac{1}{576}$ or $\frac{1}{92}$.

The number above the line is called the *numerator* and it tells us how many of the parts stated in the denominator are being dealt with in that particular instance. Hence, in the fraction $\frac{3}{4}$, something has been divided into four parts and we are dealing with only three of those parts. Similarly in the fraction $\frac{1}{1000}$ there are one thousand parts but only one of them is of immediate concern.

Dividing 1 pint into 20 parts produces 20 fluid ounces, so that 1 fluid ounce can be expressed as $\frac{1}{20}$ of a pint. If we want to express 6 fluid ounces as a fraction of a pint we first say, 'How many fluid ounces are there in a pint?' There are 20, so that becomes the denominator in the fraction. Next we say, 'How many such parts am I dealing with in this instance?' 6 such parts, so 6 is the numerator of the fraction, and we can say that 6 fluid ounces is $\frac{6}{20}$ of a pint.

Now fractions, useful as they are, have their drawbacks, and no one uses them if there is a more understandable way of expressing something. We know that there are 1000 milligrams in a gram; therefore, we usually say that a dose of such and such a medicine is 30 milligrams and not $\frac{3}{100}$ of a gram. It would be perfectly correct to say so, and under certain circumstances it might be necessary to say so, but generally speaking we prefer to use whole numbers rather than fractions. Various tables have been devised to avoid fractions.

The English systems are somewhat unwieldy and this is one of the reasons for the national policy of conversion to the more rational metric system. However, it will be a long time before the change is complete and until that day arrives we must continue to expect to have to deal with yards, feet and inches; and pints and fluid ounces. Only one good thing can be said about such systems, that is, they afford a variety of practice in fractions!

Exercises

Write as fractions:

1. Nine-sixteenths
2. Two-thirds
3. Three-sevenths
4. Ten-elevenths

Write in words:

5. $\frac{11}{20}$ $\frac{13}{14}$ $\frac{2}{3}$ $\frac{9}{17}$ $\frac{4}{9}$ $\frac{5}{12}$

Express the following as fractions of a pound (weight):

6. 1 ounce
7. 3 ounces
8. 5 ounces
9. 10 ounces
10. 8 ounces
11. 4 ounces

Express the following as fractions of a pound sterling:

12. 5p
13. 25p
14. 30p
15. 75p
16. 80p
17. 60p
18. 35p

Express the following as fractions of a metre:

19. 20 centimetres
20. 50 centimetres
21. 15 centimetres
22. 75 centimetres

Now try a few the other way round:

Find the values of:

23. $\frac{2}{5}$ of £1
24. $\frac{1}{6}$ of £3
25. $\frac{1}{4}$ of £7
26. $\frac{1}{8}$ of £2
27. $\frac{5}{8}$ of £2
28. $\frac{2}{3}$ of 1 minute
29. $\frac{11}{12}$ of 1 minute
30. $\frac{1}{5}$ of 1 metre
31. $\frac{7}{10}$ of 1 metre
32. $\frac{1}{2}$ of 1 kilometre
33. $\frac{3}{4}$ of 1 kilometre

EQUIVALENT FRACTIONS

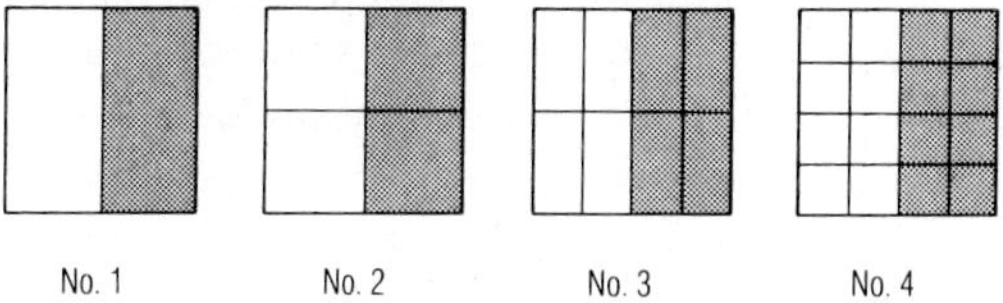

Above we have four squares of equal size. The first has been divided by a line into two halves. The second has been divided into quarters, the third into eighths, and the last into sixteenths. Look at the shaded portion in each case and you will see that half the square is shaded, but in No. 2 the shaded portion consists of two quarters, which suggests that the two quarters is the same thing as one half. Similarly, in No. 3, the shaded portion consists of four eighths, and, yet again, in No. 4, the shaded half consists of eight sixteenths. In other words we can say from this illustration that $\frac{1}{2}$ is the same as $\frac{2}{4}$ or $\frac{4}{8}$ or $\frac{8}{16}$. They are all expressed in different values but they are all equal. This leads us to a very important principle: The value of a fraction remains unaltered *when the numerator and the denominator are multiplied or divided by the same number.*

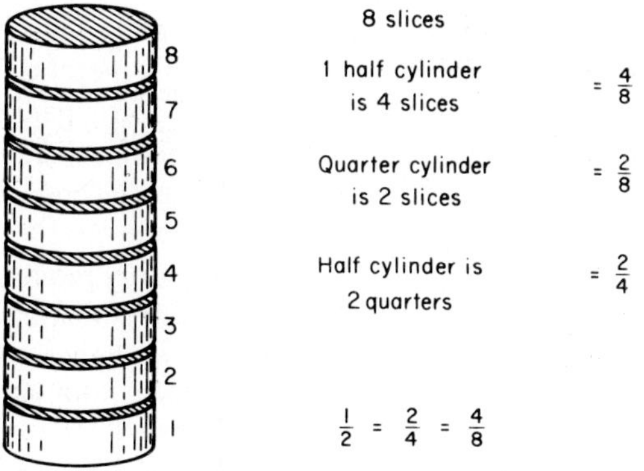

Frequently a fraction is some astronomical number that conveys no meaning whatever until it has been reduced to manageable size. For instance $\frac{40}{1000}$ is an unwieldy fraction. If we apply the above principle and divide the numerator by 2 and then the denominator by the same number, 2, the fraction becomes $\frac{20}{500}$. We can repeat the performance again and make the fraction $\frac{10}{250}$ and yet again, making it $\frac{5}{125}$. If we then divide above and below by 5 the fraction is reduced to a form that permits no further reduction, namely $\frac{1}{25}$ and we can see that $\frac{40}{1000} = \frac{1}{25}$. This process is called reducing the fraction to its lowest terms, and this is done by a process called 'cancelling' or 'cancelling out'. For brevity it is usually written as follows:

$$\frac{\overset{\overset{\overset{\overset{1}{\cancel{5}}}{\cancel{10}}}{\cancel{20}}}{\cancel{40}}}{\underset{\underset{\underset{\underset{25}{\cancel{125}}}{\cancel{250}}}{\cancel{500}}}{\cancel{1000}}} = \frac{1}{25}$$

Each division is done mentally and the result each time is entered in smaller figures and at a slightly higher level. Two things are essential when using this method. One is that each division of the numerator is accompanied by a division of the denominator by the same number, and the other is that the quotients (results of the division) must be entered neatly or confusion arises.

Cancelling in fractions is more commonly required than expanding, but it is sometimes necessary to multiply. If the following fractions are required to be arranged in increasing order of size, it can be done quite simply by observing the numerators:

$$\frac{6}{20} \quad \frac{4}{20} \quad \frac{9}{20} \quad \frac{13}{20} \quad \frac{1}{20}$$

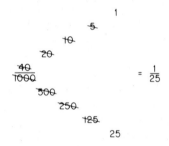

The correct order is:

$$\frac{1}{20} \quad \frac{4}{20} \quad \frac{6}{20} \quad \frac{9}{20} \quad \frac{13}{20}$$

But in the following example

$$\frac{1}{2} \quad \frac{7}{12} \quad \frac{1}{3} \quad \frac{3}{4}$$

it is not obvious at first glance which is greater or less than any of the others. It remains obscure until all the fractions are rewritten with the same denominator. Twelve is a convenient denominator for this case. To give the fraction $\frac{1}{2}$ a denominator of 12 we must multiply the denominator by 6. If we do this we must also multiply the numerator by 6. In this way $\frac{1}{2}$ becomes $\frac{6}{12}$.

Similarly by multiplying the denominator and numerator of $\frac{1}{3}$ by 4, $\frac{1}{3}$ becomes $\frac{4}{12}$. And by multiplying $\frac{3}{4}$ by 3, it becomes $\frac{9}{12}$. We can then rewrite the fractions thus:

$$\frac{6}{12} \quad \frac{7}{12} \quad \frac{4}{12} \quad \frac{9}{12}$$

and can then arrange them easily in correct size order:

$$\frac{4}{12} \quad \frac{6}{12} \quad \frac{7}{12} \quad \frac{9}{12}$$

which corresponds with

$$\frac{1}{3} \quad \frac{1}{2} \quad \frac{7}{12} \quad \frac{3}{4}$$

Later, when we come to consider the addition and subtraction of fractions, this process of multiplying up with a common denominator is essential.

Exercises

Fill in the gaps left in the following:

1. $\frac{1}{2} = \frac{5}{?} = \frac{7}{?} = \frac{?}{22} = \frac{?}{40}$

2. $\frac{3}{4} = \frac{6}{?} = \frac{12}{?} = \frac{?}{8} = \frac{?}{12}$

3. $\frac{3}{5} = \frac{?}{10} = \frac{?}{25} = \frac{21}{?} = \frac{36}{?}$

Reduce the following to their lowest terms:

4. $\frac{2}{6}$
5. $\frac{2}{10}$
6. $\frac{3}{9}$
7. $\frac{21}{28}$
8. $\frac{25}{80}$
9. $\frac{13}{52}$

In each of the following pairs, express the first part as a fraction (in the lowest terms) of the second part:

10. 6p; 12p
11. 3p; 12p
12. $7\frac{1}{2}$ milligrams; 30 milligrams
13. $1\frac{1}{2}$ milligrams; 12 milligrams
14. 10 millilitres; 1 litre
15. 20 milligrams; 1 gram
16. 1 centimetre; 1 metre
17. 50 centimetres; 1 metre
18. 750 millimetres; 1 metre
19. 30 seconds; 10 minutes
20. 40 minutes; 1 hour

FRACTIONS—WHAT THEY ARE

So far the fractions we have dealt with have all been 'proper' fractions. That is to say, that the numerators have all been smaller than the denominators, e.g. $\frac{3}{4}$, $\frac{7}{12}$, $\frac{91}{120}$. There are, however, such things as 'improper' fractions, though there is nothing wrong with them. An improper fraction is one in which the numerator is bigger than the denominator, e.g. $\frac{7}{4}$, $\frac{9}{2}$, $\frac{8}{3}$. Let us take the first of these and see what we have.

$\frac{7}{4}$ can be said 'seven-quarters', and if there are seven quarters there is enough to make 1 unit with $\frac{3}{4}$ over. Hence $\frac{7}{4}$ can be written down as $1\frac{3}{4}$.

Similarly, $\frac{5}{2}$ can be spoken of as five halves, and with five halves there is enough to make 2 whole units with $\frac{1}{2}$ over, so that $\frac{5}{2}$ can be written as $2\frac{1}{2}$.

Then again, $\frac{8}{3}$ is eight-thirds, which makes 2 whole units and $\frac{2}{3}$ over, so that $\frac{8}{3}$ can be expressed as $2\frac{2}{3}$.

Numbers that consist partly of a whole number and partly of a fraction are called mixed numbers.

5 half - litres = $2\frac{1}{2}$ litres

From this it follows that to rewrite an improper fraction as a mixed number it is necessary to divide the numerator by the denominator putting down the quotient (result of the division) as a whole number and the remainder as the fraction part.

Exercises
Try a few:
Express the following improper fractions as mixed numbers:

1. $\frac{5}{2}$
2. $\frac{5}{4}$
3. $\frac{7}{3}$
4. $\frac{8}{5}$
5. $\frac{11}{4}$
6. $\frac{48}{8}$
7. $\frac{29}{11}$
8. $\frac{18}{7}$
9. $\frac{28}{12}$
10. $\frac{32}{9}$

Conversely when it is necessary to convert mixed numbers into improper fractions, the whole-number part is multiplied by the denominator and the numerator is *added* to the product (result of the multiplication).

Example
Convert $4\frac{1}{4}$ into an improper fraction.

First, multiply the whole number, 4, by the denominator, also 4, to obtain 16. Then add the numerator, 1:

$$1 + 16 = 17$$

Therefore the improper fraction is $\frac{17}{4}$.

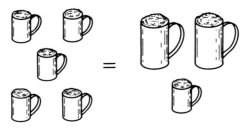

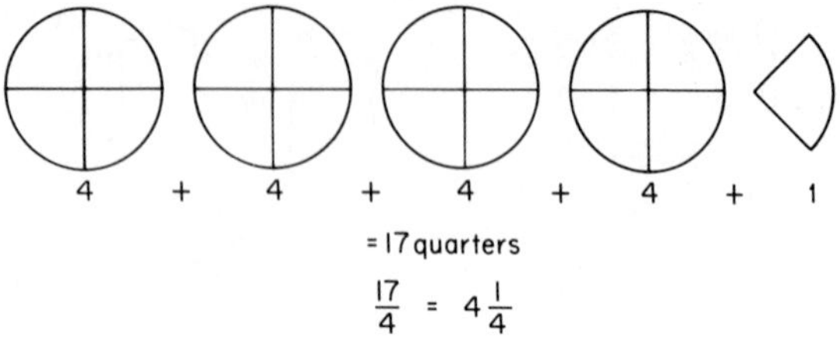

Exercises

Try these:

Express the following as improper fractions:

1. $1\frac{1}{3}$ *4.* $3\frac{1}{8}$ *7.* $3\frac{7}{10}$ *10.* $5\frac{17}{100}$

2. $1\frac{2}{3}$ 5. $4\frac{3}{8}$ *8.* $4\frac{3}{10}$

3. $2\frac{3}{4}$ *6.* $7\frac{1}{8}$ *9.* $9\frac{2}{7}$

ADDITION AND SUBTRACTION OF FRACTIONS

Add the following:

6 apples and 3 apples and 7 apples and 2 apples.

The answer is 18 apples.

Now add these:

6 apples and 3 pears and 7 oranges and 2 melons.

The proper answer is that the sum cannot be done as it stands as these are sets of different things; in other words things with different denominations. In order to do the sum they must all be of the same denomination. We can get round the difficulty only by saying that they are all fruits and therefore there are 18 fruits in all.

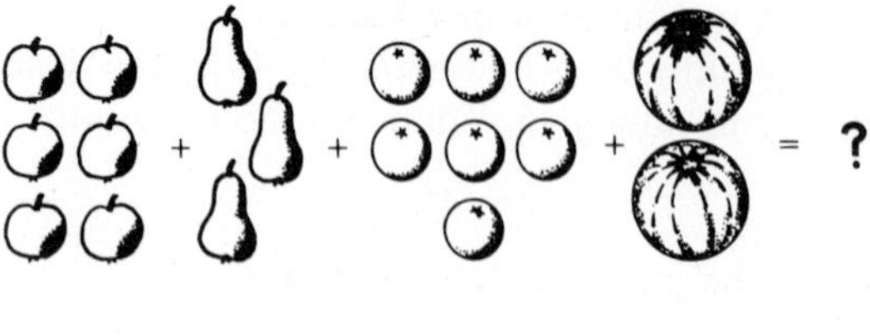

So it is with fractions.

It is easy enough to add $\frac{1}{12}$, $\frac{3}{12}$, $\frac{6}{12}$ and $\frac{7}{12}$, because they all have the same denomination, or denomin*ator* in the case of fractions. The answer is $\frac{17}{12}$ which we can condense to the mixed number $1\frac{5}{12}$.

But when we come to consider the sum of $\frac{1}{12}$, $\frac{1}{4}$, $\frac{1}{2}$ and $\frac{2}{3}$ we meet the same problem as with apples, pears, oranges and melons. These fractions all have different denominators and to make any sense out of them we must first provide them with the same denominator. This involves finding a suitable denominator and, whereas any denominator will do, it is less cumbersome to use the lowest number into which all will divide. In this case 12 is the lowest common denominator.

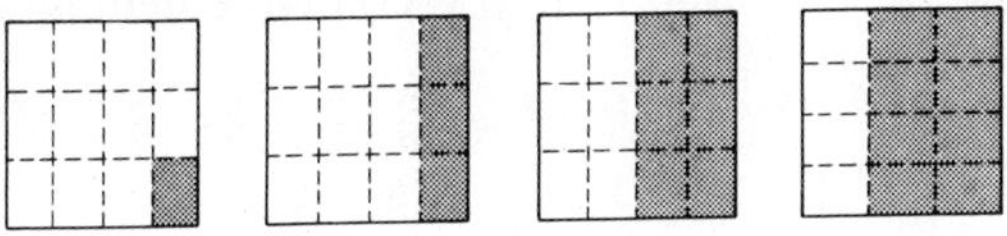

$\frac{1}{12}$ $\frac{1}{4} = \frac{3}{12}$ $\frac{1}{2} = \frac{6}{12}$ $\frac{2}{3} = \frac{8}{12}$

$\frac{1}{12} + \frac{1}{4} + \frac{1}{2} + \frac{2}{3} = \frac{18}{12}$

First we write down the sum:

$$\frac{1}{12} + \frac{1}{4} + \frac{1}{2} + \frac{2}{3}$$

Then we must take each one separately and multiply the denominator so that it is valued at 12, not forgetting that whenever we multiply a denominator we must also multiply the numerator by the same amount.

The first is already in twelfths and needs no changing.

The second, $\frac{1}{4}$, must be multipled by three above and below and becomes $\frac{3}{12}$.

The third must be multiplied by 6 above and below so that it becomes $\frac{6}{12}$.

And the last by 4 to make it $\frac{8}{12}$.

The sum can then be rewritten thus:

$$\frac{1}{12} + \frac{3}{12} + \frac{6}{12} + \frac{8}{12}$$

We can now add it very simply and it is $\frac{18}{12}$, or as a mixed number $1\frac{6}{12}$, which is the same as $1\frac{1}{2}$.

Examples
Here are three worked examples showing:

1. How an addition sum can be set out.
2. How a subtraction sum can be set out.
3. How a mixed problem can be set out.

1. Find the sum of $\frac{1}{2}$, $\frac{5}{6}$, $\frac{2}{3}$, $\frac{2}{5}$. (A suitable denominator is 30):

$$\frac{1}{2} = \frac{15}{30};\quad \frac{5}{6} = \frac{25}{30};\quad \frac{2}{3} = \frac{20}{30};\quad \frac{2}{5} = \frac{12}{30}$$

$$\begin{aligned} \therefore \frac{1}{2} + \frac{5}{6} + \frac{2}{3} + \frac{2}{5} &= \frac{15}{30} + \frac{25}{30} + \frac{20}{30} + \frac{12}{30} \\ &= \frac{72}{30} \\ &= 2\frac{12}{30} \\ &= 2\frac{2}{5} \end{aligned}$$

2. Find the value of $3\frac{1}{5} - 1\frac{2}{15} - \frac{2}{3}$. (A suitable denominator is 15):

$$3\frac{1}{5} = \frac{16}{5} = \frac{48}{15}$$

$$1\frac{2}{15} = \frac{17}{15}$$

(Converting into improper fractions)

$$\frac{2}{3} = \frac{10}{15}$$

$$\begin{aligned} \therefore 3\frac{1}{2} - 1\frac{2}{15} - \frac{2}{3} &= \frac{48 - 17 - 10}{15} \\ &= \frac{21}{15} \\ &= 1\frac{2}{5} \end{aligned}$$

3. Find the value of $4\frac{1}{4} - 2\frac{1}{8} - \frac{3}{4} + 6\frac{2}{3}$:

$4\frac{1}{4} - 2\frac{1}{8} - \frac{3}{4} + 6\frac{2}{3} = 4\frac{1}{4} + 6\frac{2}{3} - 2\frac{1}{8} - \frac{3}{4}$ (Re-arranging so that plusses come first and minuses last)

$= \frac{17}{4} + \frac{20}{3} - \frac{17}{8} - \frac{3}{4}$ (Converting to improper fractions)

(24 is a convenient common denominator)

$$\frac{17}{4} = \frac{102}{24}$$
$$\frac{20}{3} = \frac{160}{24}$$
$$\frac{17}{8} = \frac{51}{24}$$
$$\frac{3}{4} = \frac{18}{24}$$
$$= \frac{102 + 160 - 51 - 18}{24}$$

$$\therefore 4\frac{1}{4} - 2\frac{1}{8} - \frac{3}{4} + 6\frac{2}{3} = \frac{193}{24} = 8\frac{1}{24}$$

Exercises

Here are some exercises involving addition, subtraction and the finding of lowest common denominators:

1. $\frac{1}{3} + \frac{5}{9}$
2. $\frac{1}{8} + \frac{5}{8}$
3. $\frac{8}{9} - \frac{2}{9}$
4. $\frac{3}{4} - \frac{1}{4}$
5. $\frac{1}{2} + \frac{1}{5}$
6. $\frac{1}{4} + \frac{3}{5}$
7. $\frac{3}{4} - \frac{2}{3}$
8. $\frac{5}{6} + \frac{2}{9}$
9. $1 - \frac{2}{7}$
10. $\frac{7}{8} + \frac{5}{16}$
11. $\frac{3}{5} + \frac{3}{10} + \frac{1}{2}$
12. $\frac{1}{2} + \frac{1}{4} - \frac{3}{8}$
13. $\frac{3}{7} - \frac{1}{4} + \frac{1}{14}$
14. $\frac{2}{3} + \frac{7}{10} - \frac{4}{15}$
15. $\frac{4}{5} - \frac{17}{25} + \frac{1}{3}$

MULTIPLICATION OF FRACTIONS

When two or more fractions are to be multiplied together the numerators are multiplied together separately from the denominators and then all the denominators are multiplied. For example, in the expression $\frac{3}{4} \times \frac{1}{2}$, the numerators 3 and 1 are first multiplied giving a product of

3, and 3 becomes the new numerator. Next the denominators 4 and 2 are multiplied giving a product of 8. This becomes the new denominator, so that the new fraction is $\frac{3}{8}$.

$$\frac{3}{4} \times \frac{1}{2} = \frac{3 \times 1}{4 \times 2} = \frac{3}{8}$$

A half of three-quarters is three-eighths

It might be said that multiplying by a fraction is an absurdity, because the very word 'multiply' implies that as a result of the multiplication there will be more than there was formerly. Yet, from the foregoing example, it can be said that as a result of 'multiplying' by $\frac{1}{2}$ there is less than there was originally. If the expression had asked, 'What is $\frac{1}{2}$ of $\frac{3}{4}$?', it would have been both logical and correct. To cover this point mathematicians have arranged a convention, a sort of poetic licence, to regard the word 'of' in such expressions as meaning the same as would a multiplication sign. In this way such problems as the following can be written in mathematical terms:

There are 40 patients in a ward. Three-quarters *of* these are confined to bed but $\frac{2}{3}$ *of* the bed patients are allowed to wash themselves. How many bowls will be required for their use?

$$\text{Number of bowls required} = 40 \times \tfrac{3}{4} \times \tfrac{2}{3}$$

$$= \frac{\overset{10}{\cancel{40}} \times \overset{1}{\cancel{3}} \times 2}{\underset{1}{\cancel{4}} \times \underset{1}{\cancel{3}}}$$

$$= \frac{10 \times 1 \times 2}{1 \times 1}$$

$$= 20$$

Where whole numbers are concerned in the multiplication of fractions, they should be regarded as fractions with a denominator of 1, since the rule of multiplying only numerators together and only denominators together can then be applied.

Examples
Multiply $\frac{3}{5}$ by 2:

$$\begin{aligned}\tfrac{3}{5} \times 2 &= \tfrac{3}{5} \times \tfrac{2}{1}\\ &= \frac{3 \times 2}{5 \times 1}\\ &= \tfrac{6}{5}\\ &= 1\tfrac{1}{5}\end{aligned}$$

Cancelling can help to simplify the multiplication of fractions. In order to multiply $\frac{5}{12}$ by $\frac{12}{25}$, numerators must be multiplied together and so must denominators, arriving at a fraction of $\frac{60}{300}$. This is not in its simplest form, however, and to simplify, one would have to divide numerator and denominator first by twelve and then by five, reducing it to $\frac{1}{5}$. How unnecessary it would be to multiply by twelve and then divide by twelve in the next step. Cancelling will solve the problem. Set the work out thus:

$$\tfrac{5}{12} \times \tfrac{12}{25} = \frac{5 \times 12}{12 \times 25}$$

Cancelling can then proceed. Twelve in the top line and twelve in the bottom line are both divisible by twelve. Five in the top line and twenty-five in the bottom line are both divisible by five, so the expression will look like this after cancellation:

$$\frac{\overset{1}{\cancel{5}} \times \overset{1}{\cancel{12}}}{\underset{1}{\cancel{12}} \times \underset{5}{\cancel{25}}} = \frac{1 \times 1}{1 \times 5} = \frac{1}{5}$$

Next, simplify $\frac{6}{35} \times \frac{14}{15}$:

$$\frac{6}{35} \times \frac{14}{15} = \frac{\overset{2}{\cancel{6}} \times \overset{2}{\cancel{14}}}{\underset{5}{\cancel{35}} \times \underset{5}{\cancel{15}}}$$

(6 in the numerator and 15 in the denominator divisible by 3; 14 and 35 divisible by 7)

$$= \frac{2 \times 2}{5 \times 5} = \frac{4}{25}$$

Exercises

Simplify:

1. $\frac{1}{2} \times \frac{1}{4}$
2. $\frac{3}{4} \times \frac{1}{4}$
3. $\frac{3}{8} \times \frac{2}{3}$
4. $\frac{7}{8} \times 2$
5. $\frac{4}{9} \times 3$
6. $\frac{5}{6} \times \frac{1}{5}$
7. $4 \times \frac{1}{4}$
8. $\frac{1}{3} \times \frac{4}{5}$
9. $\frac{3}{7}$ of 4
10. A quarter of 2 litres

In all the above exercises only simple fractions have been used. When the fraction is a mixed number, i.e. partly a whole number and partly fraction as in $2\frac{1}{2}$, it must be converted into an improper fraction before work starts. This is different from questions involving addition and subtraction where, it will be remembered, the whole-number parts could be dealt with separately. Hence in the expression $2\frac{1}{2} + 3\frac{3}{4} - 1\frac{3}{8}$, the whole number part resulted in 4, and the fraction parts in $\frac{7}{8}$.

In multiplication the fractions must be rewritten as improper fractions, so that using the same fractions the expression is $2\frac{1}{2} \times 3\frac{3}{4} \times 1\frac{3}{8}$. Re-written it becomes:

$$\frac{5}{2} \times \frac{15}{4} \times \frac{11}{8}$$

The rule of multiplying numerators together and denominators together can then be used, and it becomes:

$$\frac{5 \times 15 \times 11}{2 \times 4 \times 8}$$

$$= \frac{825}{64}$$

$$= 12\tfrac{57}{64}$$

Here, again, cancelling can simplify the working to a considerable extent, but in the above expression there were no factors common to both the numerator and the denominator, so no cancelling could be done.

Examples
Simplify $3\frac{1}{5} \times 3\frac{5}{8} \times 1\frac{6}{29}$

$$= \frac{16}{5} \times \frac{29}{8} \times \frac{35}{29}$$

$$= \frac{\overset{2}{\cancel{16}} \times \overset{1}{\cancel{29}} \times \overset{7}{\cancel{35}}}{\underset{1}{\cancel{5}} \times \underset{1}{\cancel{8}} \times \underset{1}{\cancel{29}}}$$

$$= \frac{2 \times 1 \times 7}{1 \times 1 \times 1}$$

$$= 14$$

Cancelling has taken all the extensive multiplying and dividing out of the work. Twenty-nine was divisible by 29 in both numerator and denominator. So were 16 by 8 and 35 by 5.

Next, simplify $\frac{3}{4} \times 3\frac{1}{7} \times 11\frac{4}{11} \times \frac{1}{5} \times 7$

$$= \frac{3}{4} \times \frac{22}{7} \times \frac{15}{11} \times \frac{1}{5} \times \frac{7}{1}$$

$$= \frac{3 \times \overset{1}{\cancel{\overset{2}{\cancel{22}}}} \times \overset{3}{\cancel{15}} \times 1 \times \overset{1}{\cancel{7}}}{\underset{2}{\cancel{4}} \times \underset{1}{\cancel{7}} \times \underset{1}{\cancel{11}} \times \underset{1}{\cancel{5}} \times \underset{1}{1}}$$

$$= \frac{3 \times 1 \times 3 \times 1 \times 1}{2 \times 1 \times 1 \times 1 \times 1}$$

$$= \frac{9}{2}$$

$$= 4\tfrac{1}{2}$$

Exercises

Simplify:

1. $\frac{2}{7} \times 3$
2. $\frac{4}{9} \times 5$
3. $\frac{5}{12} \times 6$
4. $\frac{7}{8} \times 4$
5. $\frac{5}{14} \times 2$
6. $\frac{9}{15} \times 5$
7. $\frac{2}{5} \times 10$
8. $\frac{5}{28} \times 21$
9. $\frac{2}{7} \times \frac{3}{5}$
10. $\frac{4}{11} \times \frac{3}{8}$
11. $\frac{3}{4}$ of 8
12. $\frac{3}{4}$ of $\frac{8}{9}$
13. $\frac{1}{3}$ of 6
14. $\frac{1}{3}$ of $\frac{3}{4}$
15. $3\frac{1}{3} \times 6$
16. $4\frac{2}{3} \times 1\frac{1}{5}$
17. $9\frac{5}{11} \times \frac{11}{13}$
18. $2\frac{1}{5} \times 3\frac{1}{2} \times 13\frac{1}{3}$
19. $\frac{11}{81} \times 5\frac{1}{4} \times 3\frac{3}{7}$
20. $1\frac{5}{28} \times \frac{35}{36} \times 3\frac{3}{11}$

DIVISION OF FRACTIONS

It has been observed that a whole number can be written in fraction form by supplying it with a denominator of 1. For example, 2 in fractional form becomes $\frac{2}{1}$, 6 becomes $\frac{6}{1}$, 8 becomes $\frac{8}{1}$ and so on. This device is convenient when dealing with division in fractions.

If the fractional form of a number is turned upside down so that its denominator becomes its numerator and vice versa, the new fraction is called the *reciprocal* of the original fraction. For instance, 3 can be written $\frac{3}{1}$, and its reciprocal is $\frac{1}{3}$. The same is true of proper fractions. The reciprocal of $\frac{2}{7}$ is $\frac{7}{2}$; of $\frac{3}{4}$ is $\frac{4}{3}$; of $\frac{1}{2}$ is $\frac{2}{1}$. This brings us to the rule to apply when dividing by a fraction: *when dividing by a fraction convert the divisor into its reciprocal and multiply by it instead.* In more familiar language the rule can be stated thus: in order to divide by a fraction, turn it upside down and multiply by it. For example, in the expression $\frac{1}{3} \div \frac{2}{5}$, two-fifths is the divisor. Turned upside down it becomes $\frac{5}{2}$ and the expression can be rewritten as:

$$\frac{1}{3} \times \frac{5}{2}$$

It is then straightforward and equals $\frac{5}{6}$.

There is nothing more than this to the division of fractions except that mixed numbers must be changed to improper fractions before work starts.

Example
Simplify $3\frac{1}{3} \div 7\frac{2}{3}$:

$$\begin{aligned} 3\tfrac{1}{3} \div 7\tfrac{2}{3} &= \tfrac{10}{3} \div \tfrac{23}{3} \\ &= \tfrac{10}{3} \times \tfrac{3}{23} \\ &= \frac{10 \times \overset{1}{\cancel{3}}}{\underset{1}{\cancel{3}} \times 23} \\ &= \tfrac{10}{23} \end{aligned}$$

Next, divide $8\frac{1}{4}$ by $1\frac{1}{2}$:

$$\begin{aligned} 8\tfrac{1}{4} \div 1\tfrac{1}{2} &= \tfrac{33}{4} \div \tfrac{3}{2} \\ &= \tfrac{33}{4} \times \tfrac{2}{3} \\ &= \frac{\overset{11}{\cancel{33}} \times \overset{1}{\cancel{2}}}{\underset{2}{\cancel{4}} \times \underset{1}{\cancel{3}}} \\ &= \frac{11 \times 1}{2 \times 1} \\ &= 5\tfrac{1}{2} \end{aligned}$$

Exercises

Simplify:

1. $\frac{5}{6} \div \frac{3}{4}$	5. $\frac{15}{16} \div \frac{5}{4}$	9. $\frac{2}{3} \div \frac{3}{4}$
2. $\frac{4}{7} \div \frac{8}{9}$	6. $\frac{7}{8} \div 3$	*10.* $4\frac{1}{3} \div 3\frac{1}{4}$
3. $5 \div \frac{10}{11}$	*7.* $4\frac{3}{4} \div 5\frac{1}{2}$	*11.* $18 \div 1\frac{2}{7}$
4. $7 \div \frac{3}{5}$	*8.* $\frac{8}{15} \div \frac{4}{5}$	*12.* $2\frac{1}{2} \div 3\frac{1}{8}$

13. If a nurse's stride measures $\frac{3}{5}$ metre how many steps must she take to walk from the sluice to the duty room—a distance of 18 metres?

14. Sister is to buy rolls of crepe paper at $17\frac{1}{2}$p each. How many can she get for £2.60? How much money is left over and how many Christmas tree decorations at 5p each will this buy?

15. A nurse sends $\frac{1}{10}$ of her month's salary home, spends $\frac{1}{30}$ of it on a new textbook, pays $\frac{1}{5}$ to her insurance agent, and banks $\frac{1}{4}$. If she then has £85 left, what is her monthly salary?

4 Decimals

In infant schools children are taught to write down numbers under certain headings—thousands, hundreds, tens and units. Later they dispense with the headings but it is worthwhile recalling them and seeing what relationship they bear to each other. The number 6000 is spoken of as *six thousand*. Dividing it by ten results in a quotient of *six hundred*. Further division by ten results in sixty, which by continued use over centuries is a contraction of *six tens*, and a final division by ten results in *six units*. In the early days of a child's education this is as far as he may be taken and it is sufficient to show that each classification is ten times as great as its right-hand neighbour. Decimal notation is a means of continuing this system to include smaller numbers than units. A dot called the *decimal point* is placed after the units column and numbers are continued to the right of this point, each number representing one-tenth of the value of the numbers in the column on its immediate left, in the following manner:

Thousands Hundreds Tens Units (point)
Tenths Hundredths etc.

If the units 'six' are divided by ten the quotient is six-tenths, which we have seen in the chapter on fractions can be represented by $\frac{6}{10}$. It can be represented in decimals as point six, which is written .6; or more usually as 0.6, the zero being used to emphasize the decimal point and not standing for anything in particular. Without the zero the point might quite easily be overlooked.

If point six stands for $\frac{6}{10}$, division by ten would result in *six-hundredths*. The fractional form of this, $\frac{6}{100}$, is familiar but it can also be written as 0.06, the figure six now being entered in the next space after the tenths column. The process can be repeated indefinitely providing successively thousandths next to the hundredths, then ten-thousandths, then hundred-thousandths and so on.

In this way a concise method of writing down numbers without the use of denominators has been evolved. For example, the expression twenty-five, eight-tenths, seven-hundredths, three-thousandths, can be written as 25.873, and this is usually read as 'twenty-five *point* eight, seven, three'.

DECIMALS INTO FRACTIONS

The reverse process of converting decimals to fractions takes only a moment. The decimal figures are regarded as the numerator of the fraction and a denominator is supplied consisting of 1 followed by as many noughts as there are decimal figures in the numerator.

$$46{\cdot}3 = 46\frac{3}{10}$$

One decimal place, therefore 1 zero in the denominator as 3 is in the position of the tenths

$$8{\cdot}65 = 8\frac{65}{100}$$

Two decimal places, therefore 2 zeros in the denominator

$$37{\cdot}715 = 37\frac{715}{1000}$$

Three decimal places, therefore 3 zeros in the denominator

Sometimes there may be no whole number. For instance, the decimal 0.873 becomes $\frac{873}{1000}$; there being 3 figures in the numerator to the right of the decimal point, there must be three zeros in the denominator. Once the fraction has been discovered it may be necessary to cancel in order to present it in its lowest form.

Now regard the decimal 0.0004. It shows that there are no tenths, hundredths or thousands, but there are four ten-thousandths which can be written as $\frac{4}{10000}$. At first glance the rule of making the decimal the numerator with as many zeros in the denominator as there are figures in the decimal may seem to have broken down, but it has not done so. The *complete* numerator should consist of all the figures to the right of the decimal point, zeros included, namely 0004. Here there are four figures, so there should be four zeros in the denominator. Once the fraction has been calculated the zeros in the numerator are dispensed with.

Example

Convert each of the following to fractions reduced to their lowest terms:

(*a*) 3.1 $= 3\frac{1}{10}$

(*b*) 4.6 $= \dfrac{\overset{3}{\cancel{6}}}{\underset{5}{\cancel{10}}} = 4\frac{3}{5}$

(*c*) 7.45 $= 7\dfrac{\overset{9}{\cancel{45}}}{\underset{20}{\cancel{100}}} = 7\frac{9}{20}$

(*d*) 0.05 $= \dfrac{\overset{1}{\cancel{5}}}{\underset{20}{\cancel{100}}} = \frac{1}{20}$

(*e*) 17.875 $= 17\dfrac{\overset{\overset{7}{\cancel{35}}}{\cancel{875}}}{\underset{\underset{8}{\cancel{40}}}{\cancel{1000}}} = 17\frac{7}{8}$

Exercises

Convert each of the following decimals into fractions in their lowest terms:

1. 5.2	*5.* 0.06	*8.* 2.55
2. 2.5	*6.* 0.006	*9.* 1.05
3. 3.25	*7.* 4.125	*10.* 0.0005
4. 0.6		

FRACTIONS INTO DECIMALS

The reverse procedure of converting fractions to decimals is achieved by dividing the numerator of the fraction by its denominator. Hence to convert the fraction $\frac{1}{2}$ to a decimal, certain thoughts pass through one's head like this:

'Two into 1 won't go. Put a zero in the units column followed by a decimal point. Multiply the numerator by 10 by adding a zero to it. That makes the numerator 10. Divide this number by the denominator. Two into 10 goes 5 times, with no remainder. Place the 5 next to the decimal point. Therefore $\frac{1}{2} = 0.5$.'

Examples

Express $\frac{3}{4}$ as a decimal.

(Four into 3 won't go, so put down zero followed by the decimal point.)

$$0.$$

(Multiply the numerator by 10 and divide the result by the denominator: $30 \div 4$. This goes 7 times with a remainder of 2. Place the 7 in the first decimal place.)

$$0.7$$

(Multiply the remainder by 10 and divide this by the

denominator: 20 ÷ 4 = 5. Place the 5 in the next decimal place.)

$$0.75$$

$$\therefore \tfrac{3}{4} = 0.75$$

Express $\frac{3}{8}$ as a decimal:

$$\begin{array}{rll} 3 \div 8 & \text{won't go} & 0. \\ 30 \div 8 & = 3 \text{ with 6 over} & 0.3 \\ 60 \div 8 & = 7 \text{ with 4 over} & 0.37 \\ 40 \div 8 & = 5 \text{ with no remainder} & 0.375 \\ \therefore \tfrac{3}{8} & = 0.375 & \end{array}$$

Express $\frac{7}{8}$ as a decimal:

(The working can be done most conveniently in the margin as a simple or long division sum.)

$$\tfrac{7}{8} = 0.875$$

Exercises

Express each of the following fractions in decimal form:

1. $\frac{7}{20}$
2. $\frac{3}{25}$
3. $\frac{5}{16}$
4. $\frac{33}{40}$
5. $\frac{9}{32}$
6. $\frac{53}{80}$
7. $2\frac{13}{20}$
8. $3\frac{15}{32}$
9. $\frac{113}{40}$
10. $\frac{432}{125}$

RECURRING DECIMALS

It is quite impossible to convert some fractions to complete decimals. For instance, in the fraction $\frac{1}{3}$, the process of dividing by three after multiplying each remainder by ten results in a series of quotients of 3, and always there is another remainder of 1. The decimal would look like this:

0.33333333333333333333.... with 1 remaining

These are called *recurring* decimals, and to indicate that such is the case a dot is placed over the number that recurs, thus 0.3. It occurs in many fractions, particularly those with a denominator of 3, 6, 7, 9.

An interesting type of recurrence occurs with decimals derived from any fraction with a denominator of 7. Instead of a single figure recurring, a whole set does so in regular order:

$$\frac{1}{7} = 0.142857142857142857 \ldots$$
$$\frac{2}{7} = 0.2857142857142857 \ldots$$
$$\frac{3}{7} = 0.42857142857142857 \ldots$$
$$\frac{4}{7} = 0.5714285714285714285 7 \ldots$$
$$\frac{5}{7} = 0.71428571428571428 57 \ldots$$
$$\frac{6}{7} = 0.857142857142857142857 \ldots$$

It can be seen that the recurring block consists of the figures 142857. In such a case recurrence is denoted by placing a dot over both the first and last figures of the recurring block as in $\frac{4}{7} = 0.57\dot{1}4285\dot{7}$.

Such decimals can be a great nuisance in mathematics and where they occur they are best left as fractions if it is possible to do so. A fraction is always complete and exact whereas a recurring decimal is an approximation. Fortunately recurring decimals rarely occur in nursing problems.

MULTIPLICATION IN DECIMALS

1. Copy the expression carefully onto some paper.
2. Add up the total number of decimal places in the numbers as written in rule (1).
3. Work out a rough answer using approximate values of the numbers instead of decimals.
4. Ignore the decimal points and multiply the numbers as if they were ordinary whole numbers.

5. Write down the product as a whole number.
6. Starting at the right-hand figure in the product as written under rule (5) count as many figures as there are decimal places under rule (2).
7. Place the decimal point in front of that many figures.
8. Check with the rough answer made in rule (3) to see if the answer is feasible.

These rules will be clearer if a few examples are worked.

Examples

Simplify 0.5 × 3.2:

1. 0.5 × 3.2
2. There is a total of two decimal places, one from the 0.5 and one from the 3.2.
3. (Rough answer 0.5 × 3 = 1.5)
4. 5 × 32
5. = 160
6. Starting with the right-hand figure, count two places and insert the decimal point to the left of the second, 1.60
7. Check with the rough answer to make sure that the answer is feasible. (In this case the final zero can be omitted once the position of the decimal point has been established, but not before.)

Simplify 7.46 × 3.2 × 14.7:

Rough answer 7 × 3 × 15 = 315

746 × 32 × 147	(This may be worked by long multiplication in the margin.)
= 3501984	(Decimal places total 4, two from 7.46, one from 3.2, and one from 14.7. Therefore the decimal point is placed in front of the fourth figure from the right.)
350.9184	(Which agrees with the rough answer.)

Multiply together 2.9, 0.58, 1.03:
Rough answer $3 \times 0.5 \times 1 = 1.5$
$29 \times 58 \times 103 = 173246$ (5 decimal places)

1.73246

Sometimes the product of two or more decimals does not contain enough figures to apply the rule for the correct placing of the decimal point. In such a case enough figures are created by placing zeros to the left of the figures in the product. For instance 0.5×0.005 gives a product of 25 and the decimal point must be placed in front of the fourth figure. Obviously there are only two figures in 25, but by placing two zeros in front of them there will be no alteration in their value but it will then be possible to place the decimal point in its correct place: 0.0025.

Multiplying decimals by 10 merely involves shifting the decimal place one position to the right. For instance, 5×10 as everyone knows is 50. If we express 5 as 5.0 it will be seen that in the product, the decimal point has moved one place to the right. Similarly, right throughout decimals this is possible:

$$0.005 \times 10 = 0.05$$

When multiplying by 100 the decimal point is moved two places to the right. This is quite clear if 100 is looked upon as consisting of 10×10. Multiplying by 10 involves moving the decimal one place to the right, therefore multiplying twice by 10 involves moving the decimal two places to the right.

Multiplying by 1000 involves three shifts to the right as 1000 equals $10 \times 10 \times 10$, and so on.

In this fact lies the beauty of the metric system in which all measurements are in units that have one-tenth of the value of the next highest measure. 1 decimetre is $\frac{1}{10}$ of a metre, 1 milligram is $\frac{1}{10}$ of a centigram, etc.

Exercises

1. Multiply each of the following by 10:
(*a*) 0.7 (*b*) 1.7 (*c*) 0.007 (*d*) 3.04 (*e*) 7.32

2. Multiply each of the following by 100:
(*a*) 3.2 (*b*) 17.04 (*c*) 0.007 (*d*) 1.007 (*e*) 13.1

3. 4.83 × 0.3
4. 37.4 × 0.5
5. 2413 × 0.04
6. 0.73 × 0.8
7. 3.142 × 0.7
8. 0.83 × 1.1
9. 0.83 × 0.11
10. 8.3 × 0.011
11. 0.077 × 0.03
12. 3.24 × 8.46
13. 37.4 × 0.05483
14. 7.5 × 0.75 × 0.075
15. 92 × 0.31 × 2.3
16. 36.9 × 1.014 × 2.5

DIVISION IN DECIMALS

Consider the following expression: 'Three divided by four'. This can be written in fractional form $\frac{3}{4}$ as has been seen in the chapter on fractions. Similarly, the expression: 'Point five divided by point two five' can be written in fractional form:

$$\frac{0.5}{0.25}$$

It will be remembered that fractions can be expanded by multiplying both the numerator and the denominator by equal amounts. The resulting fraction may not look anything like the original, but it has exactly the same value. This principle can be used to great advantage when dealing with expressions such as that written above.

$$\frac{0.5}{0.25} \text{ looks ugly}$$

If the numerator and the denominator are multiplied by 100 it becomes $\frac{50}{25}$. It looks nothing like the original but we know it has the same value and is a much more manageable expression. Clearly 50 divided by 25 equals 2.

It is only necessary to convert the denominator into a whole number. The denominator is the number that is going to be used to do the dividing and is called a *divisor*. If this is in whole-number form the division can progress in the margin in simple or long form, whichever is most convenient, even if the numerator still has a decimal point in it. Hence, the expression:

'divide 1.326 by 0.3'

when rewritten in fractional form becomes

$$\frac{1.326}{0.3}$$

Multiplying top and bottom by 10 makes it a simple division sum:

$$\frac{13.26}{3} = 4.42$$

A rule for the division of decimals can now be formulated.

To divide by a decimal, rewrite the expression as a fraction and multiply the numerator and the denominator by a number sufficient to convert the denominator into a whole number.

It is wise not to omit rewriting the expression as a fraction until the multiplication is fully grasped, but that step can be left out once confidence has been gained.

Examples

Divide 17.943 by 0.25

$$= \frac{17.943}{0.25} \text{ (multiply top and bottom by 100)}$$

$$= \frac{1794.3}{25}$$

$$= 71.772$$

Simplify $0.072 \div 0.0012$

$$= \frac{0.072}{0.0012} \text{ (multiply top and bottom by 10000)}$$

$$= \frac{720}{12}$$

$$= 60$$

Divide 27.42 by 0.032

$$= \frac{27.42}{0.032} \text{ (multiply top and bottom by 1000)}$$

$$= \frac{27420}{32}$$

$$= 856.875$$

Exercises

1. Express as decimals or whole numbers:

(*a*) $0.45 \div 0.5$	(*f*) $5.0008 \div 89.3$
(*b*) $0.44 \div 1.1$	(*g*) $0.76107 \div 0.23$
(*c*) $0.32 \div 0.08$	(*h*) $0.0032 \div 0.08$
(*d*) $0.0066 \div 0.6$	(*i*) $12.63 \div 0.3$
(*e*) $12 \div 0.04$	(*j*) $25 \div 0.5$

2. Multiply each of the following by 10, 100, 1000:
(*a*) 9.9 (*b*) 8.79 (*c*) 0.6 (*d*) 0.01 (*e*) 0.65
(*f*) 0.408 (*g*) 93.28 (*h*) 7.05 (*i*) 40.02

3. Divide each of the following by 10, 100, 1000:
(*a*) 750 (*b*) 62.32 (*c*) 4.23 (*d*) 0.025

4. Write as decimals:
   (*a*) $\frac{72}{10}$ (*b*) $\frac{93}{100}$ (*c*) $\frac{12}{1000}$ (*d*) $\frac{7008}{100}$
5. Express the following decimals in fractional form in their lowest terms (or as mixed numbers where appropriate):
   (*a*) 0.9 (*b*) 0.09 (*c*) 0.25 (*d*) 2.25
   (*e*) 0.448 (*f*) 2.076 (*g*) 0.0025
6. Simplify each of the following expressions:
   (*a*) 2.5×0.023 (*b*) 0.006×1.08 (*c*) 32.75×4.8 (*d*) 11.81×4.2 (*e*) 39.44×2.3 (*f*) 4.29×61.12
7. Express as recurring decimals:
   (*a*) $\frac{1}{3}$ (*b*) $\frac{5}{6}$ (*c*) $\frac{1}{9}$ (*d*) $\frac{3}{11}$ (*e*) $\frac{1}{7}$
8. Express the following to three significant figures:
   (*a*) 24 780 (*b*) 275 999 (*c*) 975 900
   Express the following to two significant decimal places:
   (*d*) 0.00758 (*e*) 0.8768 (*f*) 0.0939 (*g*) 0.06717

5 The Metric System

Opinion in favour of adopting the metric system in preference to the older English systems of measurement gradually gained strength during the first half of this century. It was argued that there were many advantages to be obtained from using the same methods of measurement that are used by most other countries. This has become particularly important as closer economic, social and political links have been established between the United Kingdom and Western Europe.

There is also much to commend the discarding of lengthy and poorly understood methods for simpler ones, provided there is no loss of efficiency. Such views were held by the rulers of France at the end of the eighteenth century, for it was they who introduced the metric system into Europe in a successful bid to simplify matters. In that era there were not merely a few units of measurement to confuse the populace, there were no fewer than 200 standards of weight alone and no matter how conservative one's views may be it is obvious that such a state of affairs could not have been allowed to continue.

In 1790 an invitation was extended from France to this country to share in a common metric system of weights and measures, but no action was taken here. However, in Europe and elsewhere the metric system gained rapid acceptance. An international treaty, the Metric Convention, was signed by 17 countries in 1875, and by the United Kingdom in 1884. More than 90% of the world's people are now using the metric system of measurement.

Following a request from the Federation of British Industries in 1965 the Government finally agreed to introduce the metric system; 1975 was set as the target date for completion of the changeover. To assist in the changeover the Metrication Board was set up in 1969, but for a variety of reasons the target date was not achieved, although the metrication of the pound sterling, with the abolition of shillings and pennies and the introduction of new pence each worth £$\frac{1}{100}$, had taken place in 1971.

Official adoption of the metric system by the National Health Service for handling pharmaceutical preparations was an important step in the process of metrication. Once nurses became accustomed to administering medicines in metric doses they quickly realized that the metric system is easier to understand than traditional English weights and measures.

There is one basic unit for each property to be measured such as weight or volume. The size of a unit can be expressed in terms of multiples of tens or tenths of other units. Thus, expression of measurements in terms of higher or lower units becomes easy as only an adjustment of the decimal point is required. Moreover, the units are based on some definite, measurable and fixed standard and not, as previously, on some variable and ill-defined quantity like the length of an arm from elbow to finger-tip, or the weight of a grain of wheat.

The unit of length is the metre. The standard for this measurement is the length of a bar of platinum–iridium kept at the International Bureau of Weights and Measures at Sèvres in France at a temperature of 0°C. More accurately it has been defined as the wavelength of an orange line in the krypton spectrum.

The unit of volume is the litre, which is equal to the volume of a cube measuring 1 decimetre along each edge, that is 1 cubic decimetre or 1000 cubic centimetres.

The unit of weight is the kilogram. The standard for this is the weight of a cylinder of platinum–iridium, which is also kept at Sèvres. It is approximately equal to the weight of 1000 cubic centimetres of water at 4°C at sea level.

Multiples of the basic measurements occur in steps of ten. The same principle applies to fractions of the base unit. A prefix indicates the enhanced or diminished value of the basic unit.

Prefix	*Factor*	*Symbol*
mega	one million times	M
kilo	one thousand times	k
hecto*	one hundred times	h
deca*	ten times	da
deci*	one-tenth	d
centi*	one-hundredth	c
milli	one-thousandth	m
micro	one-millionth	μ

The prefixes marked * are not normally used in everyday matters. The accepted symbols are shown above, but it is always wise to write terms in full whenever an error could lead to serious consequences. Consideration of the symbols M and m; k and h; da and d; clearly reveals the danger of not writing symbols legibly, if they are to be used at all.

Using these prefixes, tables are built up as follows:

Distance

10 millimetres (mm)	= 1 centimetre	(cm)
10 centimetres	= 1 decimetre	(dm)
10 decimetres	= 1 *metre*	(m)
10 metres	= 1 decametre	(dam)
10 decametres	= 1 hectometre	(hm)
10 hectometres	= 1 kilometre	(km)

Weight

10 milligrams (mg)	= 1 centigram	(cg)
10 centigrams	= 1 decigram	(dg)
10 decigrams	= 1 *gram*	(g)
10 grams	= 1 decagram	(dag)
10 decagrams	= 1 hectogram	(hg)
10 hectograms	= 1 kilogram	(kg)
1000 kilograms	= 1 tonne	(t)

The accepted symbol for a gram in prescription writing is G. In all other cases the international symbol g should be used. The word 'gram' was formerly written as 'gramme' except when accompanied by a prefix or when used in writing prescriptions (to avoid confusion with the word 'grain').

Area

100 square millimetres	= 1 square centimetre	(cm^2)
100 square centimetres	= 1 square decimetre	(dm^2)
100 square decimetres	= 1 *square metre*	(m^2)
100 square metres	= 1 square decametre	(dam^2)
100 square decametres	= 1 square hectometre	(hm^2)
100 square hectometres	= 1 square kilometre	(km^2)

The *are* is the unit for measuring the area of land. Thus:

100 square metres	= 1 are	(a)
100 ares	= 1 hectare	(ha)

Volume

1000 cubic millimetres (mm^3)	= 1 cubic centimetre	(cm^3)
1000 cubic centimetres	= 1 cubic decimetre	(dm^3)
1000 cubic decimetres	= 1 cubic metre	(m^3)

Different terms are used to describe measurement of capacity, although these are linked to volume as shown below.

Capacity

10 millilitres (ml)	= 1 centilitre	(cl)
10 centilitres	= 1 decilitre	(dl)
10 decilitres	= 1 *litre*	(l) = 1 cubic decimetre (dm^3)
10 litres	= 1 decalitre	(dal)
10 decalitres	= 1 hectolitre	(hl)

The international symbols have been shown and the danger of confusing these with one another will again have been noticed. It cannot be stressed too strongly that terms should be written in full whenever the consequences of error would be serious.

Measuring the very small

Many substances used in medicine in these modern times have to be measured in exceedingly small doses. To eliminate the use of fractions and decimals the prefixes micro; nano; pico; femto; and atto have been introduced. The first of these prefixes is the only one likely to be needed by nurses. For example, a microgram is one-thousandth of a milligram (0.000001 g). It can be abbreviated to μg (the Greek letter mu), but this looks so similar to mg for milligram that it is often wiser to write it in full.

Similarly microscopic distances are better expressed in whole numbers rather than decimal points followed by strings of zeros. Thus a micron is one-thousandth of a millimetre, which, if you have a ruler graduated in centimetres and millimetres before you, you will agree is an exceedingly small distance. One of the smallest micro-organisms visible through an ordinary microscope is the virus of smallpox which is about 0.2 microns (micrometres, μm), in diameter. Red blood cells are about 7 microns in diameter and about 2 microns in thickness. See how much easier it is to say and write this than to say that red blood cells are 0.007 mm in diameter and 0.002 mm in thickness.

Exercises

Complete the following sums:

1. 1 g = ... mg
2. 1 litre = ... ml
3. 3155 mm = ... m
4. 250 ml = ... litre
5. 1500 mg = ... g
6. 1.75 litre = ... ml
7. 50 ml = ... litre
8. 1.08 litre = ... ml
9. 0.062 g = ... mg
10. 960 ml = ... litre
11. 45.9 ml = ... litre
12. 9.6 kg = ... g
13. 40 litres + 364 ml = ... litre
14. 32 mg + 760 mg + 480 mg = ... g
15. 8 litres − 469 ml = ... litre .... ml
16. 0.54 mg + 920 mg + 663 mg − 1.56 g
= .... mg = ... g
17. 0.75 mg = ... μg
18. 750 microns = ... mm

Conversion from one scale to another

All hospitals are now using metric measurements and, gradually, they are being introduced into everyday life. However, the public will take some considerable time to adjust to the method, and to begin to think in grams instead of pounds. It will, therefore, still be necessary for nurses to translate for their patients, and to be able to convert from one system to another. Instances of this could be with the measuring of diets, such as those for diabetics who have to weigh the ingredients, or for mothers who cannot understand the instructions on a tin of infant milk powder.

Usually it is impossible to state exactly what a unit in one scale is in terms of the units of another. The best that can be achieved is an approximation. For instance, one can state that a metre equals 39.4 inches. For most everyday purposes this would be quite adequate, but if one wanted greater accuracy one could use the figure of 39.37, or closer still—39.369, or even 39.3693. In other words it is possible to go on adding decimal places making the approximation closer and closer but never arriving at a figure which is the exact equivalent of 1 metre. It is the same with all other such conversion figures.

The important question in all conversions from one scale into another is, 'How accurate must I be?' If a nurse were asked to measure a patient's leg for the fitting of a caliper and to give the measurement in metric units, she might, if she were unwise, measure with an inch tape measure and then convert to metres by using the conversion figure of 39.3693. This would give an answer that would be very exact but would be more exact than the makers of the caliper could work to. As the accuracy of the apparatus is rarely closer than the nearest tenth of an inch the nurse need merely have used the conversion figure of 39.4, thus saving herself much mental effort and reducing the risk of error considerably.

In all the following paragraphs a working conversion figure is given. This should be adequate for almost all conversions met within the ordinary course of events in the wards. Given in brackets is a more accurate figure which can be used if a very close approximation is required.

MEASURES OF LENGTH

Inches and centimetres

1 inch (in) = $2\frac{1}{2}$ centimetres (cm) (2.54 cm)

To convert inches to centimetres multiply by $\frac{5}{2}$
To convert centimetres to inches multiply by $\frac{2}{5}$

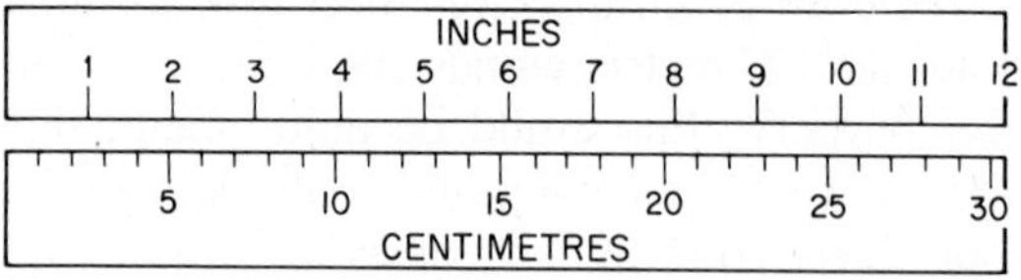

The degree of accuracy achieved with this figure is within one-fifth of an inch for every foot. For example:

12 inches = $12 \times \frac{5}{2}$
= 30 centimetres using the $2\frac{1}{2}$ conversion figure
12 inches = 12×2.54
= 30.48 centimetres using the 2.54 conversion figure

Hence there is undervaluation of nearly $\frac{1}{2}$ a centimetre which is almost exactly one-fifth of an inch. It would be wise, therefore, to add one-fifth of an inch to every foot when converting to centimetres and to subtract that amount for every 30 centimetres when converting to inches.

Millimetres and inches

1 millimetre = $\frac{1}{25}$ inch (0.039 in)

To convert millimetres to inches multiply by $\frac{1}{25}$
To convert inches to millimetres multiply by 25

Measurement of blood pressure is usually expressed in millimetres of mercury. This is explained fully in Chapter 15.

To get a clear picture of the length of a millimetre take an ordinary ruler that is graduated in metric units along one edge. Usually there is a blank stretch about 4 inches long. This is a decimetre, which is one-tenth part of a metre. Decimetres are not used very much. Next there is another decimetre divided into ten sections, each of which is a centimetre. Next, each centimetre is divided into ten equal sections and each one is a millimetre.

Examples

How many millimetres must be cut from a sheet of paper 21 centimetres long to make it fit into a book 6 inches long?

$$\begin{aligned} \text{6 inches} &= 6 \times 25 \text{ mm} \\ &= 150 \text{ mm} \\ \text{21 cm} &= 210 \text{ mm} \\ \therefore \text{ length to be removed} &= 210 - 150 \text{ mm} \\ &= 60 \text{ mm} \end{aligned}$$

A measurement has been expressed as '5 inches'. Express this in millimetres.

$$\begin{aligned} \text{5 inches} &= 5 \times 25 \text{ mm} \\ &= 125 \text{ mm} \\ \therefore \text{ the measurement} &= 125 \text{ mm} \end{aligned}$$

MEASURES OF WEIGHT

Kilograms and pounds

1 kilogram (kg) = $2\frac{1}{5}$ pounds (lb) (2.205 lb)

To convert kilograms to pounds multiply by $\frac{11}{5}$
To convert pounds to kilograms multiply by $\frac{5}{11}$

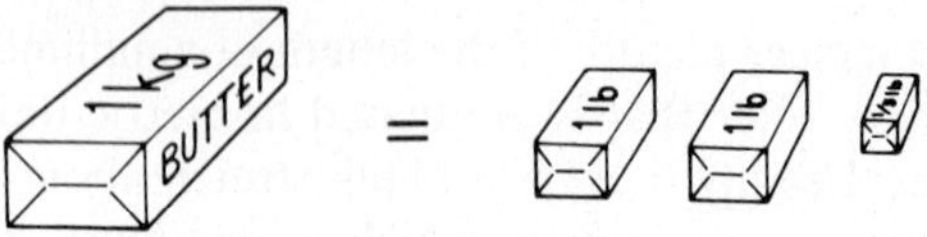

1 kilogram = $2\frac{1}{5}$ pounds

Examples

If a patient weighs 65 kg what is this in stones and pounds?

$$\begin{aligned} 65 \text{ kg} &= 65 \times \tfrac{11}{5} \text{ lb} \\ &= 13 \times 11 \text{ lb} \\ &= 143 \text{ lb} \\ &= 10 \text{ st } 3 \text{ lb} \end{aligned}$$

What is 1 cwt in kilograms?

$$\begin{aligned} 1 \text{ cwt} &= 112 \text{ lb} \\ &= 112 \times \tfrac{5}{11} \text{ kg} \\ &= \tfrac{560}{11} \text{ kg} \\ &= 51 \text{ kg approximately} \end{aligned}$$

(The ‘round figures’ 1 cwt = 50 kg are often used for quick calculation.)

MEASURES OF VOLUME

Litres and fluid ounces

1 litre (l) = 35 fluid ounces (fl oz) (35.196 fl oz)

To convert litres to fluid ounces multiply by 35
To convert fluid ounces to litres multiply by $\frac{1}{35}$

Examples

A pint of water weighs $1\frac{1}{4}$ lb. What does a litre weigh in ounces (Avoirdupois)?

$$1 \text{ pint} = 20 \text{ fl oz}$$
$$= \overset{4}{\cancel{20}} \times \frac{1}{\underset{7}{\cancel{35}}} \text{ litres}$$
$$= \tfrac{4}{7} \text{ litres}$$

$\therefore \frac{4}{7}$ of a litre weighs $1\frac{1}{4}$ lb
$\therefore$ 1 litre weighs $1\frac{1}{4} \times \frac{7}{4}$ lb

$$= \frac{5}{\underset{1}{\cancel{4}}} \times \frac{7}{\underset{1}{\cancel{4}}} \times \overset{\overset{1}{\cancel{4}}}{\cancel{16}} \text{ oz } (1 \text{ lb} = 16 \text{ oz})$$
$$= 35 \text{ oz}$$

If an arm bath is to contain 5 litres of saline and you have only a pint measure, how much will you measure out?

$$5 \text{ litres} = 5 \times 35 \text{ fl oz}$$
$$= \frac{\overset{1}{\cancel{5}} \times 35}{\underset{4}{\cancel{20}}} \text{ pints}$$
$$= \tfrac{35}{4} \text{ pints}$$
$$\therefore = 8\tfrac{3}{4} \text{ pints}$$

$\therefore$ you would measure out $8\frac{3}{4}$ pints

Exercises

1. Convert each of the following to (i) kilograms, (ii) pounds:
(*a*) 0.5 g × 450 (*b*) 177.5 g × 20
(*c*) 6.5 g × 34 (*d*) 400 g × 3.5

2. Express each of the following in (i) kilograms, (ii) grams:
(Work to 3 decimal places only.)
(*a*) $\frac{1}{2}$ lb (*b*) 10 lb (*c*) 2.2 lb (*d*) $5\frac{1}{2}$ lb.

3. In a class, six of the pupils weigh 40, 48, 56, 58, 62 and 100 kg.
   (*a*) Express each of these weights in stones and pounds.
   (*b*) What is the average weight of these six in kilograms and in pounds?
4. Calculate the total quantity of the following drugs consumed by an average of ten people, for each drug, in (i) millilitres and (ii) litres:
   (Doses given are for one person.)
   (*a*) Potassium citrate (BNF) 10 ml, three times daily for 5 days.
   (*b*) Aluminium hydroxide mixture 5 ml three times a day for 3 weeks.
   (*c*) Chloral hydrate (BNF) 20 ml once a day for 2 weeks.
5. (*a*) Express the following in pints and fluid ounces:
   40 ml 100 ml 1.5 litres 500 ml 375 ml
   (*b*) Express the following in litres or millilitres:
   1 pint 2 fl oz $\frac{1}{2}$ fl oz
6. The daily dosage of streptomycin is expressed as 20 milligrams per kilogram of body weight. What would the dosage be for a man weighing 60 kilograms?
7. Arrange the following in size order of weight:
   1086 mg 0.75 kg 1 lb 0.8 g
8. Arrange the following in size order of volume:
   0.5 litre 0.75 pint 180 fl oz 625 ml 300 cc
9. If 4.5 litres of milk is supplied to a 20-bed ward, how much is allowed per patient? Express the answer in (*a*) litres, (*b*) decilitres, (*c*) millilitres.
10. How many trays with an area of 0.75 square metres can be laid on a table with an area of 17.25 square metres?
11. If a bank pays £2.50 interest on each £100 deposited for 1 year, how much interest will a nurse get who

Table 1. Millimetres to inches and inches to millimetres

Millimetres	*Inches*	*Inches*	*Millimetres*
1000	40	100	2500
900	36	90	2250
800	32	80	2000
700	28	70	1750
600	24	60	1500
500	20	50	1250
400	16	40	1000
300	12	30	750
200	8	20	500
100	4	10	250
90	3.6	9	225
80	3.2	8	200
70	2.8	7	175
60	2.4	6	150
50	2.0	5	125
40	1.6	4	100
30	1.2	3	75
20	0.8	2	50
10	0.4	1	25
9	0.36	0.9	22.5
8	0.32	0.8	20
7	0.28	0.7	17.5
6	0.24	0.6	15
5	0.2	0.5	12.5
4	0.16	0.4	10
3	0.12	0.3	7.5
2	0.08	0.2	5
1	0.04	0.1	2.5

Table 2. Kilograms to Pounds and Pounds to Kilograms

Kilograms	*Pounds*	*Pounds*	*Kilograms*
100	220	100	45.4
90	198	90	40.9
80	176	80	36.3
70	154	70	31.8
60	132	60	27.2
50	110	50	22.7
40	88	40	18.2
30	66	30	13.6
20	44	20	9.1
10	22	10	4.5
9	19.8	9	4.1
8	17.6	8	3.6
7	15.4	7	3.2
6	13.2	6	2.7
5	11	5	2.3
4	8.8	4	1.8
3	6.6	3	1.4
2	4.4	2	0.9
1	2.2	1	0.45

leaves £270.32 in the bank for 3 years? (Simple interest)

12. The analysis written on a patent food packet states
0.7 parts carbohydrate
0.25 parts protein
0.05 parts fat
What weight of each is present in a 500-gram packet?

CONVERSION TABLES

Tables 1 to 3 are ready reckoners which make conversion much easier. They contain, however, approximate conversions only and therefore the answers obtained from

Table 3. Millilitres to Fluid Ounces and Fluid Ounces to Millilitres

Millilitres	*Fl ounces*	*Fl ounces*	*Millilitres*
1000	35	10	285
900	31.5	9	257
800	28	8	228
700	24.5	7	200
600	21	6	172
500	17.5	5	143
400	14	4	114
300	10.5	3	86
200	7	2	57
100	3.5	1	28
90	3.1	0.9	26
80	2.8	0.8	23
70	2.5	0.7	20
60	2.1	0.6	17
50	1.8	0.5	14
40	1.4	0.4	11
30	1.1	0.3	9
20	0.7	0.2	6
10	0.35	0.1	3

them are not very accurate, particularly when comparatively large numbers are being converted. To use them, split the amount to be converted into hundreds, tens, units and decimals and look up each of these separately; then add the answers for each.

For example, to convert 174 inches into millimetres, look up the figures for 100 inches then for 70 and then 4, and add all these together:

100 inches= 2500 mm
70 inches= 1750 mm

$$4 \text{ inches} = 100 \text{ mm}$$
$$\therefore 174 \text{ inches} = 4350 \text{ mm}$$

Before these tables are used to convert parts of a whole, it will be necessary to change the amount to be converted, if it is expressed as a vulgar fraction, into a decimal fraction, e.g. $\frac{1}{5}$ inch = 0.2.

Exercises

1. Convert each of the following to inches:
(*a*) 946 mm (*b*) 33 mm (*c*) 128 mm
(*d*) 37 mm (*e*) 85 mm (*f*) 1263 mm
(*g*) 21 mm (*h*) 14 mm (*i*) 178 mm

2. Convert each of the following to millimetres:
(*a*) 42 in (*b*) 88 in (*c*) $1\frac{3}{4}$ in (*d*) $22\frac{1}{2}$ in (*e*) 38 in
(*f*) 2.9 in (*g*) 14.6 in (*h*) 56.8 in (*i*) 72 in

3. A certain film star's measurements are 36 in, 22 in, 35 in. How might this be expressed in France?

4. Convert the following to pounds:
(*a*) 65 kg (*b*) 132 kg (*c*) 48 kg (*d*) 21 kg (*e*) 106 kg
(*f*) 33 kg (*g*) 76 kg (*h*) 16 kg (*i*) 52 kg

5. Convert the following to kilograms:
(*a*) 74 lb (*b*) 153 lb (*c*) 33 lb (*d*) 92 lb (*e*) 64 lb
(*f*) 39 lb (*g*) 66 lb (*h*) 68 lb (*i*) 21 lb

6. The following are the weights of patients. Convert them to metric units:
(*a*) 7 st 12 lb (*b*) 8 st 2 lb (*c*) 10 st 6 lb (*d*) 14 st
(*e*) 13 st 7 lb (*f*) 15 st

7. A patient is told he is 1 st 4 lb overweight. How much is this in kilograms?

8. The doctor orders 4 mg of a drug per kg of body weight to be given. If the patient weighs 156 lb, how much drug is he given in mg?

9. Convert the following to fluid ounces:
(*a*) 530 ml (*b*) 220 ml (*c*) 1910 ml (*d*) 830 ml (*e*) 640 ml
(*f*) 320 ml (*g*) 750 ml (*h*) 550 ml (*i*) 470 ml

10. Convert the following to millilitres:
(*a*) 53 fl oz (*b*) 28 fl oz (*c*) 33 fl oz (*d*) 4.6 fl oz
(*e*) 15 fl oz (*f*) 4.1 fl oz (*g*) 32 fl oz (*h*) 9.6 fl oz
(*i*) 83 fl oz

6 Percentages

If the words 'per cent' are translated, they mean 'in each hundred' and for this the symbol '%' is often used. The uncertainty that may arise in the mind when the words per cent are met with can usually be removed if it is remembered that they mean simply 'in each hundred' or 'in every hundred'. Thus, if it is said that 52% of the English population is female it means that 52 people *in every hundred* are female. We may also say that 85% of the world's population have Rhesus positive blood, or that 30% of urban children are Mantoux positive by the age of 15 years.

This method of expression is so concise and convenient that it is one of the favourite tools of the statistician. Indeed it is becoming so common, particularly in American semi-scientific accounts, that it is being used increasingly as a joke by stage comedians!

One of the great advantages of the percentage system is that it gives people a small, easily managed figure that can be used as a yardstick for making comparisons, where the actual figures would convey little or nothing. For example, if we take the unemployment figures for the United Kingdom in the early 1960s we see that approximately 300 000 people were unemployed in a population of about 40 million. 300 000 is approximately $\frac{3}{4}$% of that number. In the winter of 1976 the number of unemployed people had increased to nearly $1\frac{1}{2}$ million in a population that had increased to over 50 million. Thus the percentage had increased to nearly 3%. By 1981 the actual figure was 3 million and from this you will be able to estimate the percentage of the population involved. In cases such as this the use of percentages permits direct comparisons to be made.

The greatest use made of percentages in the everyday work of a nurse is in strengths of liquid solutions. We are all conversant with such things as sodium citrate $2\frac{1}{2}\%$, cocaine 1%, surgical spirit 70%, chlorhexidine 5% and others. In all such cases, the actual quantities used may be

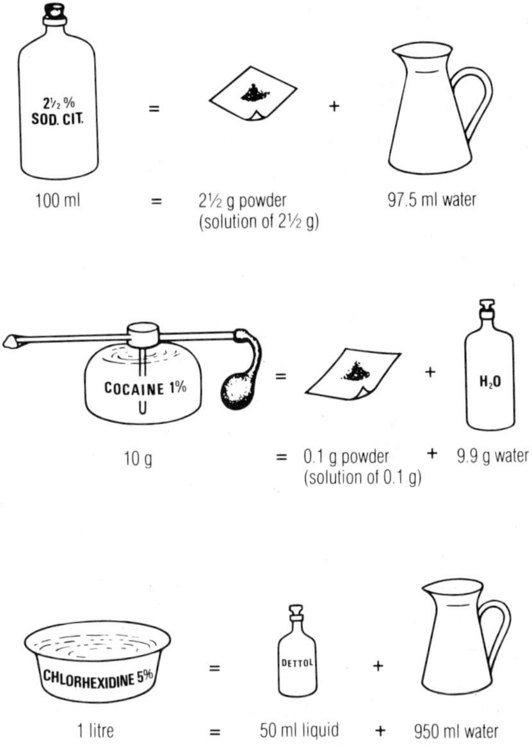

of little account. The strength is what matters, and whether one has 1 millilitre or 1 litre of a 1% solution, it remains a 1% solution. To find out exactly how much of a particular substance (the 'active principle'), is present takes only a moment if the strength is known, and also the total quantity one is dealing with. For instance, to find out how much pure chlorhexidine is present in a litre of solution of 5% strength, one says to oneself: 'In a 5% solution there are 5 parts of pure chlorhexidine in every 100 parts of solution. If there were 100 litres of solution it would contain 5 litres of chlorhexidine. If there were 100 millilitres it would contain 5 millilitres. Therefore I can say that five-hundredths ($\frac{5}{100}$) of any quantity of 5% solution will be the amount of pure substance contained in that particular quantity. Hence $\frac{5}{100}$ of a litre is the amount of pure chlorhexidine in 1 litre of 5% strength.

Five-hundredths of a litre is an unwieldy measure. It is far better to express it in millilitres. This involves a little arithmetic and one continues thus: 'There are 1000 millilitres in a litre. Therefore $\frac{5}{100}$ of a litre is 50 millilitres:

$$\frac{5}{\underset{1}{\cancel{100}}} \times \overset{10}{\cancel{1000}} = 50$$

Therefore, in every litre of chlorhexidine 5% there are 50 millilitres of pure chlorhexidine.

By similar reasoning one can work out such questions as, 'How much pure substance is required to make a particular quantity of solution of a particular strength, or how much can be made with a certain quantity?'

We have seen enough of fractions and decimals to know that they are interchangeable. So too with percentages. If 10% represents 10 parts in 100 parts, it is the same thing as the fraction $\frac{10}{100}$, which in its simplest terms is $\frac{1}{10}$. This, in its turn, is the same as 0.1. Similarly:

$$3\% \text{ is the same as } \frac{3}{100} \text{ or } 0.03$$

$$17\% \text{ is the same as } \frac{17}{100} \text{ or } 0.17$$

$$14.8\% \text{ is the same as } \frac{14.8}{100} \text{ or } 0.148$$

Therefore it is true to say that *any percentage figure can be written in fractional form by placing the percentage figure down as the numerator with 100 as the denominator.* In other words—divide the percentage figure by 100.

The converse of this is that *any fraction can be written as a percentage figure by multiplying the fraction by 100:*

$$\begin{aligned} \tfrac{3}{4} &= \tfrac{3}{4} \times 100\% \\ &= \tfrac{300}{4} \\ &= 75\% \end{aligned}$$

The rules for converting decimals to percentages and vice versa are similar. *Any percentage figure can be written in decimal form by dividing the figure by 100:*

$$\begin{aligned} 75\% &= 75 \div 100 \\ &= 0.75 \end{aligned}$$

Conversely, *any decimal fraction can be written in percentage form by multiplying the decimal by 100:*

$$\begin{aligned} 0.25 &= 0.25 \times 100\% \\ &= 25\% \end{aligned}$$

Expressing things in percentage form is a convenient and short method which applies to any quantity which, expressed in actual concrete units, would have to be different in each individual case. For instance, if one determines that one will save some money each month, it is a much better idea to decide that a certain percentage shall be banked, say 5% or 10% than to fix on a definite quantity, say £10. In this way the amount saved will vary with the income each month. If there have been a lot of deductions leaving less than is usual, one is faced with banking a smaller amount and one's resolve is not embarrassed by having to deduct yet another £10 from a slim income. On the other hand, when one's salary is swollen with bonus, income tax rebate or emoluments for holiday periods, one has the satisfaction of seeing a larger quantity than £10 tucked safely away. The concrete amount varies from month to month but still remains 5% whether it is on £10 or £10 million.

To work out the concrete sums takes only a few moments. Simply multiply the amount by the percentage figure and divide by 100.

Examples

If it has been agreed that 5% of the beds available in a small town will be kept vacant for sudden emergencies, how many beds are so reserved if there is a total bed list of 400?

Multiplying the total beds available by the percentage figure and dividing by 100 gives us this expression:

$$\frac{400 \times 5}{100} = 20$$

$\therefore$ there are 20 beds reserved.

How much chlorhexidine in its pure state is required to make 9 litres of 1% solution?

$$\frac{9 \times 1}{100} = \frac{9}{100}$$

$$= 0.09 \text{ litre}$$

$$0.09 \text{ litre} = 90.0 \text{ millilitres}$$

If simple interest is paid by a loan club at the rate of $2\frac{1}{2}\%$ per annum, how much interest is paid on £45 in 2 years?

$$\text{Interest in 1 year is } \frac{£45 \times 2\frac{1}{2}}{100}$$

In 2 years it is twice this

$$= \frac{£45 \times 2\frac{1}{2} \times 2}{100}$$
$$= £45 \times \tfrac{5}{2} \times 2 \times \tfrac{1}{100}$$
$$= £\tfrac{9}{4}$$
$$= £2\tfrac{1}{4}$$
$$= £2.25$$

Exercises

1. Convert each of the following percentages to (i) fractions, and (ii) decimals:
(*a*) 1% (*b*) 10% (*c*) 15% (*d*) 20%
(*e*) 40% (*f*) 50% (*g*) 75% (*h*) 90%

2. Convert each of the following fractions to percentages:
(*a*) $\frac{1}{100}$ (*b*) $\frac{1}{20}$ (*c*) $\frac{6}{25}$ (*d*) $\frac{7}{20}$
(*e*) $\frac{81}{900}$ (*f*) $\frac{24}{25}$ (*g*) $\frac{3}{4}$ (*h*) $\frac{7}{8}$

3. Rewrite each of the following decimals as percentages:
(*a*) 0.3 (*b*) 0.75 (*c*) 0.42 (*d*) 0.01
(*e*) 0.66 (*f*) 0.25 (*g*) 0.305 (*h*) 0.393

4. If 25% of a class of 32 nurses have a negative reaction to the Heaf test, how many should receive BCG?

5. How much pure ammonia is in a bottle containing 300 ml of strong ammonia solution if it is a 40% solution?

6. How much pure chlorhexidine is required to make 2 litres of 10% dilution?

7. A nurse gets 40 marks out of 60 in a test. Express this as a percentage.
8. If 25% of the proceeds from a sale of work is sent to the Hospital League of Friends, how much is sent if the sale nets £84.52?
9. If 15% of the patients in a hospital of 400 are under 18 years of age, how many adults are there?
10. Calculate the superannuation payable to a retiring nurse if she is to get 40% of her salary annually and has been getting £12500.00 per annum.

7 An Introduction to Chemistry

During recent years the work of a nurse has changed very considerably. At one time the number of drugs available was very limited, as was the range of surgical and medical treatments. Nowadays the situation has greatly changed; new drugs which have been made synthetically by chemists are produced almost daily and patients require highly complex treatments such as dialysis, assisted ventilation and specialized intravenous therapy. It is necessary for the nurse to assist with these and to have an understanding of the procedures, and for this reason it is essential to possess some basic knowledge of chemistry. Furthermore, now that S.I. units have been introduced, the nurse will be able to understand the terminology only after learning some chemical terms.

A book such as this cannot attempt to discuss in any depth a subject as wide as chemistry, but can merely provide a brief introduction in order to familiarize the nurse with some of the facts which she will come to be aware of during the course of her normal duties.

Chemists are involved in the study of Matter. This can be defined as a substance which occupies space, which can be divided, and which possesses weight. The chemists attempt to purify the various substances by which they are surrounded in the world and to analyse their component parts. When they have done this, they can work out how all the parts combine together to form a substance such as, for instance, glucose.

Like most subjects, chemistry has become highly specialized. The branch with which nurses are concerned is known as biochemistry and involves the study of the subject as it relates to living things. As techniques have become more refined and knowledge has increased, it has become possible to introduce more sophisticated treatments for those who are sick. Whether or not these treatments are being effective is frequently monitored by the hospital biochemists, and all nurses know that most patients quickly accumulate note folders of amazing thickness which are very largely filled with the results of laboratory investigations. In fact, although most people would be reluctant to admit it, all human metabolism is a series of chemical reactions and when any of these does not take place correctly, a person becomes ill.

Many people feel that chemistry is a subject which is far too difficult for them to understand, because of its intangibility. Forming a concept of molecules is difficult, and so the whole subject becomes complicated. All explanations here will therefore be kept as simple as possible, and any reader who wishes to obtain further information should refer to a standard textbook.

Atoms and elements

All chemical compounds are formed by the combination of two or more *elements*. There are about one hundred elements; they cannot be split into simpler substances by chemical means, nor can they be converted into each other. The elements are represented by symbols, e.g. C for carbon, H for hydrogen, O for oxygen. Elements, however, are composed of small particles, and the smallest of these are *atoms*. Atoms also consist of smaller particles, but it is only necessary to mention one type, the *electron*.

When two or more elements join to form a compound,

As we have already seen, certain atoms are able to combine with others and form molecules or compounds. Some atoms combine with one other, some with two and so on. This ability to combine is known as the valency of that atom, and once again, hydrogen is taken as the one with which this ability is compared, since it has the lowest combining power of all atoms.

Atoms which can combine only with one other are said to be *monovalent,* those which can combine with two are termed *divalent*, and so on. Hydrogen is monovalent, as are sodium and chlorine which combine with each other to form sodium chloride (NaCl). Oxygen is divalent and so by combining with two molecules of hydrogen forms water (H_2O).

The relevance of this may be appreciated when reading the results of electrolyte tests of patients. It can be seen that although the results are given in millimoles per litre, some of the figures are the same as the previous ones. This is because these atoms are monovalent, and were previously estimated as the amount per litre, so no further simplification was necessary. Only when more complex substances with atoms of greater valency are being analysed does the figure change.

It is hoped that this brief explanation of some basic chemical terminology will assist in understanding the next chapter on S.I. units.

Further reading

MacAlpine, Bruce G. (1966) *Teach Yourself Chemistry.* London: English Universities Press.
Rose, Steven (1970) *The Chemistry of Life.* Harmondsworth: Pelican.

it means that the atoms of these have combined to form a *molecule*. Thus one atom of sodium (Na) and one of chlorine (Cl) combine to form a molecule of sodium chloride (NaCl).

Sometimes two atoms of the same element will combine and form a molecule. That is how oxygen is formed, O_2.

Atomic and molecular weight

Even though atoms are so small, chemists have managed to formulate a table which shows their relative weights. This is called the Periodic Table. Hydrogen is the lightest of the atoms and has been allotted an atomic weight of 1. Carbon has an atomic weight of 12 and oxygen 16. When 2 or more atoms combine to form a molecule, the atomic weight of the individual atoms can be added together to give the molecular weight.

In general the weight of the molecule increases with its complexity and some of the proteins have a molecular weight of over 1 million.

Although all this might seem very far removed from nursing, a knowledge of it becomes important when discussing, for instance, renal function. The kidneys filter substances up to a molecular weight of 68 000, which means that only the very largest particles are not filtered. It is not necessary for the nurse actually to remember individual weights, but just to be familiar with the terminology.

The combining power of atoms

The way in which atoms combine conforms to strict rules and often this is dependent on whether they are electrically charged. You may remember that atoms contain smaller or subatomic particles which are called electrons. If one of these is removed, or one added, the atom becomes charged either positively or negatively. Thus sodium, which can easily lose an electron, may become positively charged and is written Na^+. Chlorine, which is able to accept another electron, may become negatively charged, and is written Cl^-. Elements which have a positive charge are attracted to those which have a negative charge and will thus unite to form a molecule, e.g. NaCl (sodium chloride). Atoms and molecules which carry electric charges are called *ions*.

If an ionic compound is dissolved in a liquid the compound will separate into its ionic constituents; and when evaporated back out of the solution the ionic constituents will reunite. For example when sodium chloride (NaCl) is dissolved in water it *dissociates* into sodium and chloride ions (Na^+ and Cl^-); when the solution is evaporated to dryness, a white powder remains behind; the sodium and chloride ions have *associated* to form sodium chloride.

When two ions combine in the manner described the resulting compound is called a *salt*, and this frequently occurs as the result of a reaction between an acid and an alkali. All nurses are familiar with these substances and know that the one counteracts the other. An example of this can be seen when treating patients with peptic ulcers. The excessive production of hydrochloric acid (HCl) in the stomach is counteracted by the administration of an alkali.

Acid–base balance

One of the most important ways in which we all maintain life is by the control of our acid–base balance. The production of acid and alkaline substances by the body must be finely controlled and a failure of this mechanism will cause a person to become seriously ill. The balance is maintained by respiration and the functioning of the kidneys, and disease affecting either of these can cause a

disturbance of the balance. An increase in the blood leve of acid is called *acidaemia*, and of alkali *alkalaemia*.

An acid is a substance which contains hydrogen ion (H^+), and an alkali contains negative hydroxyl ion (OH^-). The level of acidity of a substance can be mea sured and is known as the pH or percentage hydroger ('hydrogen ion concentration'). The scale for measuring this has 7 as its neutral point; anything below this is acidi and anything above is alkaline.

The pH of blood must be maintained between ver narrow limits, namely 7.35 and 7.45, which is slightl alkaline. The pH of stomach contents on the other hand varies from 1.5 to 2.5.

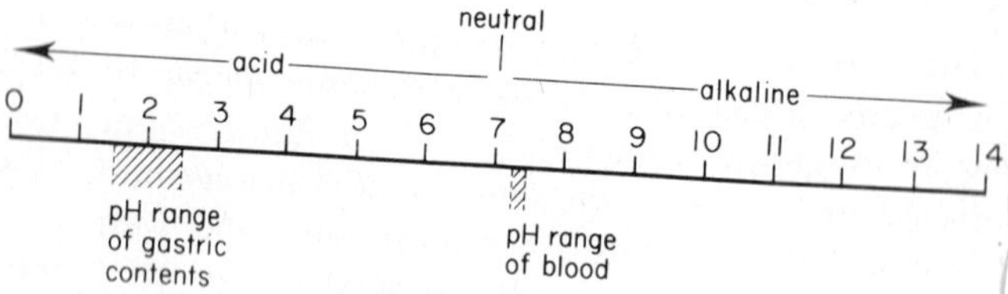

The pH scale

It has already been said that the purpose of a chapte about chemistry in a book about mathematics is to assi the reader to understand the many figures with which sh or he has to become familiar. The introduction of S units has meant a great change for nurses, particula with the use of the mole or millimole instead of mg p 100 ml. A definition of the mole is given in Chapter 8 a it is sufficient to say here that this unit is now employe describe the number of particles which are present i solution: the more concentrated a solution is, the gre the number of particles in a given volume of it. In orde understand this it is necessary to be familiar with definitions given earlier, plus one other, which is *vale*

8 S.I. Units

AN HISTORICAL INTRODUCTION

The Système International d'Unités was introduced for general use in British hospitals on 1 December 1975, despite a considerable amount of protest. The use of this new method meant that all hospital staffs had to forget the measurements and symbols with which they were familiar, and learn an almost new language.

The history of this system dates back to the early part of this century. After the adoption of the metric system it was found, in the early 1900s, that the three original basic units of length, mass and time, namely the centimetre, the gram and the second, were inadequate, particularly in the field of physics which was at that time progressing very rapidly. Because of this, three more units were added, and these were the metre, the kilogram and the ampere.

Fifty years later the system was again found to be inadequate to deal with the vast increase in scientific knowledge which had been acquired during this century, probably a greater increase than at any time in our history. It was therefore decided that a system was required which would encompass present-day needs and, as a result, in the 1960s an international organization was established and was named the General Conference on Weights and Measures. This body revised and extended the existing system, and called it the Système International d'Unités. This is now used by scientists throughout the world, but its use in hospitals in this country has come very late. The generally accepted abbreviation for the system is S.I. units.

Many people in hospitals, including the medical staffs, argued that the adoption of S.I. units was unnecessary and that the old system worked very well. Nurses tended to adopt the attitude that the system was extremely complicated and beyond their understanding. There were many questions asked as to why yet another change was necessary, and there was some suspicion of it being a political gambit.

The introduction of S.I. units, however, completed the process of metrication, and meant that all industry and science throughout the world could employ the same 'language' for measurements. It is in fact a scientific Esperanto, and its introduction should mean that error and confusion are reduced to a minimum. In the fields of medicine, where the lives of patients are involved, this is, of course, of great importance, since treatment nowadays is frequently based on information gained from laboratory investigations the results of which are given in figures. In theory, it should mean that the results of investigations can be interpreted easily, not only in another hospital, but in another country. Until recently, a variety of systems had been used, and this created a potentially dangerous situation. The use of S.I. units should therefore cause less rather than more complications, but only if all those who are in contact with it, and who need to interpret the readings, take the time to learn and understand the method.

BASIC UNITS

The S.I. system comprises seven basic units, from which calculations can be made. These are shown in Table 4. The definitions of these units are as follows:

Table 4. The Seven Basic Units of the S.I. system

Physical quantity	*Name of unit*	*Symbol*
Mass	Kilogram	kg
Length	Metre	m
Time	Second	s
Electric current	Ampère	A
Temperature	Kelvin	K
Luminous intensity	Candela	cd
Amount of substance	Mole	mol

The kilogram (kg)
The kilogram unit is based on the weight of a cylinder of platinum–iridium which is kept in France at Sèvres, near Paris. The use of this was originally adopted in 1875.

The metre (m)
The international metre was adopted for use in 1962, and is based on the wavelength of an orange line in the krypton spectrum.

The second (s)
This unit is now based on the frequency of radiation of the caesium atom.

The ampère (A)
This unit is based on the attractive force produced when an electric current flows through two straight and parallel conductors, which are one metre apart.

The degree kelvin (K)
The degree kelvin is described in relation to degrees Celsius (centigrade). Absolute zero $0\,K = -273.15°C$. For

practical purposes, degrees Celsius will continue to be used. Body temperature, 37°C, is equal to 311 kelvin.

The candela (cd)
A candela is described as 1/60th of the luminous intensity per square centimetre of platinum at 1773°C.

The mole (mol)
A mole is described as the amount of substance which contains the same number of elementary units as there are atoms to be found in 12 grams of carbon. In practical terms a mole is the molecular weight of a substance expressed in grams. Since this unit is of great importance in medicine, further explanation will be given later in the chapter.

In addition to the seven basic units, there are a number which have been obtained or derived from a combination of these. The important ones are shown in Table 5.

Table 5. Derived Units

Physical quantity	*Name of unit*	*Symbol*
Force	Newton	N
Pressure	Pascal	Pa
Energy (work)	Joule	J
Volume	Litre	l or litre

The newton (N)
A newton is the force which will accelerate a mass of 1 kilogram by one metre a second per second.

The pascal (Pa)
The pascal is a unit of pressure which is derived by relating force to area, and results from the application of 1 newton

per square metre. This should be the unit for the recording of blood pressure, but the old method employing mmHg will continue to be used, since the expense of changing every sphygmomanometer is at the moment prohibitive. Blood gas estimations will, however, be expressed in kilopascals (kPa).

The joule (J)

The joule is described as the potential energy which is released when 1 kilogram in weight falls through 1 metre by the force of gravity. The joule should now be used as an energy unit instead of the calorie and is the measurement in which dietary requirements should be expressed. However, the metrication board decided to retain the calorie at the present time. Nevertheless it might be worth becoming familiar with the relationship between the two measurements. Since the joule is smaller than the calorie, dieticians are using the kilojoule, which is one thousand times greater.

1 calorie= 4.184 joules
and 1000 calories= 1 Calorie
1 Calorie= 4184 joules
or
1 Calorie= 4.184 kilojoules
1000 Calories= 4184 kilojoules

The litre (l)

The unit of volume is the cubic metre. This, however, is too large for use in biochemistry, and so the cubic decimetre (1000 cubic centimetres) has been substituted. The universally accepted term for this is the litre, and it will continue to be used in medicine. Most nurses are, of course, already familiar with the litre since it has been common practice to measure the fluid intake and output of patients in this way for a number of years.

The millimole

Since the introduction of S.I. units, the majority of biochemical results have been expressed in millimoles per litre, and it is this unit which has caused the greatest confusion.

It is necessary at this point to return to the definition of a mole. A mole is the molecular weight of a substance expressed in grams. For example, sodium chloride comprises one atom of sodium and one of chlorine. The molecular weight of sodium is 23 and that of chlorine 35.5. The molecular weight of sodium chloride is thus 23 + 35.5 = 58.5. A mole of sodium chloride is thus 58.5 grams.

The mole, however, is a very large unit and is impractical for use in biochemistry. As a result, the most commonly used unit in medicine is the millimole, which is one thousand times smaller. This is used for substances, such as potassium chloride, which are added to intravenous infusions, as well as for the results of laboratory investigations. Concentrations are given in millimoles/litre (mmol/litre).

If the exact molecular weight of a substance is uncertain, the molar system cannot be used. This means that the concentration of a substance has still to be expressed in grams or milligrams per litre. One such substance is serum protein which, instead of being expressed in grams per 100 ml (grams %), is now expressed in grams per litre. Thus if one has a reading of serum protein at 7 grams per 100 millilitres it will now be recorded as 70 grams per litre. Haemoglobin, which is a complex molecule, will continue to be expressed as hitherto, in grams per 100 millilitres (g/100 ml).

Many of the electrolyte readings will appear to be the same in the new units as in the old. This is owing to their chemical structure, for they are monovalent. This does at least mean that the figures for the normal values of these will remain the same, but it must always be remembered that the units in which they are being expressed are different. For instance, the normal range of plasma sodium was previously expressed as 135–143 milliequivalents and is now 135–143 millimoles/litre.

FORMULAE FOR CONVERSION

There are, of course, formulae for converting from one system to the other, and those for converting from mg/100 ml and from milliequivalents/litre to millimoles/litre are given below.

Conversion from milliequivalents/litre to mmol/litre
Firstly divide by the molecular weight to convert from mg to mmol and then multiply by 10 to convert from 100 ml to 1 litre. For instance, if the molecular weight of glucose is 180 and one wishes to convert a reading of 180 mg/100 ml, the method used is as follows:

$$180 \div 180 = 1$$
$$1 \times 10 = 10$$

$\therefore$ the concentration is 10 mmol/litre

Again, if one knows that the molecular weight of urea is 60 and one wishes to convert a reading of 60 mg/100 ml, the same principle is used:

$$60 \div 60 = 1$$
$$1 \times 10 = 10$$

So the converted readings are both the same.

Conversion from milliequivalents/litre to mmol/litre
This is a little more complicated.

$$\text{Number of equivalents} = \frac{\text{weight in grams}}{\text{equivalent weight}}$$

$$= \frac{\text{weight in grams} \times \text{valency}}{\text{molecular weight}}$$

Both these formulae require a greater knowledge of chemistry than is possessed by the majority of nurses. However, having been given them, they can be used if the molecular weight of the substance in question is known, and this can be discovered by referring to the Periodic Table.

RULES FOR THE USE OF S.I. UNITS

In order to reduce the margin of error, the General Conference on Weights and Measures stipulated the way in which the symbols should be abbreviated and written down. It was decided that the abbreviations should *not* alter in the plural. Therefore when describing weight:

One kilogram = 1 kg
Ten kilograms = 10 kg

It is incorrect to add an 's' to the symbol.

Multiples and submultiples

Multiples and submultiples are formed by using prefixes:

e.g. 1 *milli*gram= 1/1000th of 1 gram
1 *kilo*gram= 1 gram × 1000

Time

Time is always expressed in seconds, and is not converted into minutes and hours.

Decimal points

The decimal point is shown as a full-stop on the line. A raised point now indicates a multiplication sign. In addition, in Western Europe, it is acceptable to use a comma as decimal point. Thus two and a half might be written as either 2.5 or 2,5. When writing large numbers, the figures should be grouped in threes. This means that five million five hundred thousand should be written in the following way

5 500 000

with a space between the figure groups.

The number can be expressed more shortly as

$$5.5 \times 10^6 \text{ or } 5{,}5 \times 10^6$$

10^6 being 10 to the power of 6 or the number multiplied by itself 6 times.

PRACTICAL EFFECTS OF S.I. UNITS

For nurses, the most noticeable effects of the introduction of S.I. units are in the reading of biochemical results and the administration of intravenous additives. It could be argued that these are of no concern to nurses since they are the responsibility of the medical staff. This, of course, is strictly true, but the needs of patients are better served if nurses can take an intelligent interest in their welfare. It is therefore helpful if the nurse who receives a laboratory report can decide whether or not the doctor should be called immediately, and in view of this it would seem expedient for everyone to become familiar with the new system.

Most hospitals have produced their own information booklets which show the new values. Study of such books will show the difference between the old units and S.I.

units, and the dangers of confusing the two. It is hoped that, as with the conversion to decimal currency, everyone will gradually forget the old systems and learn to think entirely in the new.

Further reading

Bold, A.M. and Wilding, P. (1975) *Clinical Chemistry*. Oxford: Blackwell Scientific.

Green, J.H. (1976) *An Introduction to Medical Physiology*, 4th edition. Oxford: Oxford University Press.

9 The Mathematics of Body Fluids

There are 45 litres of water in the body of an adult person weighing 70 kg, representing between 60% and 70% of his total weight. At first this may seem to be a great deal of water, but when one considers the vast number of chemical changes that are happening in every part of the body, almost all of which depend on water, the wonder is not that there is so much but that the body is able to manage with so little. This is because the water is constantly on the move: into and out of the cells; into the digestive tract, and then back into the blood for use elsewhere; carrying waters into the kidneys, leaving them there and passing back into the blood again for other tasks; into the cerebrospinal fluid, and out again; and so on. Indeed, life itself depends on this constant movement of water. Every cell needs a regular supply of raw materials to perform its functions, and these can reach the cells only when dissolved in water. Each cell must get rid of its waste substances and its manufactured products, and these also can be transported only when dissolved in water.

The 45 litres of water in the body are divided between the cells, the tissue spaces and the plasma cells in the following amounts. That inside the cells is called the intracellular fluid and amounts to 30 litres; in the tissue spaces are 12 litres of extracellular fluid and in the plasma there are about 3 litres. In addition there are about 125 ml of water in the cerebrospinal fluid.

For these quantities to remain fairly constant, losses from the body must be balanced by intake, and in healthy people this occurs. Excessive consumption of fluids is quickly followed by increased output, and when the output causes the total quantities to fall below a certain level thirst is experienced and the loss is made good by drinking. In illness the balance is often upset and one of the major tasks of the nurse is to keep accurate records of intake and output and to try to balance these each day. In Chapter 16 the methods used to keep these records are explained.

Inside the body we find that the blood is the transport system which carries water to and from the places where it is needed. In the digestive system over 5 litres of water are secreted each day and almost all of this is reabsorbed back into the blood. About 1500 ml of saliva, 2500 ml of gastric juice, 700 ml of pancreatic juice, 500 ml of bile and 200 ml of intestinal juice are needed for the digestion and absorption of food. In order to get rid of the waste products dissolved in the blood, very large amounts of water are filtered out of it each day. About 137 litres of water pass from the blood into the kidney tubules, but almost all of this is taken back into the blood, and only about 1000 to 1500 ml leave the body each day in the form of urine. Everywhere we find the same sort of cycle, from blood to tissue fluid, from tissue fluid into the cells, and then back again to the blood via the tissue fluid or the lymph. Hence very little water is lost compared with the huge quantities that are in use. Losses occur mainly in urine, about 1000 to 1500 ml; in sweat, the amount of which is very variable but is at least 500 ml a day; from the lungs, also variable and depending on the humidity of the external air, about 400 ml; and a little in faeces and tears.

BLOOD

Blood is an extremely complex liquid consisting of 55% plasma and 45% cells. Many substances are dissolved in the plasma and as long as a person remains healthy the concentrations of these vary very little. During illness changes may occur, and it is common in hospitals nowadays for specimens of blood to be taken from patients so that the laboratory staff can analyse them and estimate the quantities of solutes that are present. In this way diagnoses can be made or confirmed, treatment can be regulated and the progress that the patient is making can be checked.

One of the tests commonly carried out is to determine the amount of glucose in the blood. This is normally between 3.5 and 6.7 mmol/litre, but in diabetes mellitus it is greater. Insulin is therefore injected to reduce the amount but there is no standard dose suitable for all diabetics. Each patient has to be stabilized on a daily dosage peculiar to his own condition and this may involve repeated examinations of the blood. If too much insulin is given the level of glucose in the blood falls dangerously low, while not enough insulin allows a gradual accumulation of glucose until it reaches dangerously high levels. Attention must be paid to the diet at the same time as insulin dosage is being established, so that the carbohydrates from which glucose is derived are kept at a constant daily intake. To balance the two, and yet to provide a nourishing and interesting diet, is a fascinating problem involving mathematics, nutrition, dietetics and biochemistry.

Another test often performed is one designed to discover the amount of blood urea. Normally there is between 3.3 and 7.0 mmol/litre of blood. Urea is a waste product derived from the metabolism of proteins and the kidneys are responsible for its removal from the blood. In kidney disease the ability to excrete urea and other protein wastes is impaired and the amount of damaged kidney tissue can be estimated by measuring the amount of urea in the blood.

Blood clotting

The ability of blood to coagulate, or clot, is not fully understood. The process involves the interaction of several substances, some of which have not yet been isolated and identified but are nevertheless thought to be present. One of the known substances needed is an enzyme called thrombin. It is not present as such in blood except as prothrombin, an inactive forerunner of thrombin. During the clotting process prothrombin is turned into thrombin, which then acts on fibrinogen to make fibres of fibrin which entrap the blood cells to form the jelly-like clot. If there is insufficient prothrombin the time needed to form a clot is extended and severe haemorrhage may occur in the meantime.

Normally there are about 40 mg of prothrombin in each decilitre (100 ml) of plasma. This figure is maintained by new prothrombin which is made in the liver, but only if there is an adequate supply of vitamin K. If there is insufficient vitamin K the blood level of prothrombin falls and then there is a danger that haemorrhage will occur. This is seen in people with obstructive jaundice or other conditions where no bile is passing into the intestines. It occurs in these cases because bile is necessary for the absorption of vitamin K. A blood test soon shows when the prothrombin level has fallen and, from this, the amount of vitamin K that will have to be injected. In some forms of hepatitis the liver cells lose their ability to make prothrombin even though there is a plentiful supply of vitamin K. The efficiency of the liver can be determined by comparing the amounts of prothrombin before and after injections of vitamin K.

In certain diseases the blood may clot inside a blood vessel. This clot is called a thrombus. In the treatment of such conditions drugs called anticoagulants are used. Two of these, dicoumarol and phenindione (Dindevan), interfere with the formulation of prothrombin and so render the blood less liable to clotting. These drugs are dangerous and their use is controlled by a careful watch on the blood level of prothrombin.

Haemoglobin

Oxygen is needed by every cell in the body tissues. It is carried to them in the red cells of the blood, which are filled with a protein substance called haemoglobin. The normal quantity of haemoglobin is about 13 to 16 grams per decilitre of blood, and 1 gram of haemoglobin combines with 1.34 ml of oxygen. Thus the amount of haemoglobin gives a good guide to the oxygen-carrying capacity. In many diseases the level of haemoglobin falls. This may or may not be accompanied by a fall in the number of red cells, depending on what is causing the anaemia. As the cause is treated the amount of haemoglobin rises to normal and may exceed this, so checks are carried out throughout the treatment. Owing to the complex nature of haemoglobin it has been agreed that the concentration in the blood will, for the time being, continue to be expressed as the mass concentration. The decilitre, however, will be used instead of 100 ml and the normal haemoglobin level, therefore, will be read as:

Men: 13.5–18.0 g/dl
Women: 11.5–16.5 g/dl

Blood cells

When a specimen of blood is taken for estimation of red- and white-cell content, the laboratory technician is faced with a long and intricate task. The normal average red-cell content of blood is 5 to 6 $\times 10^{12}$/litre; white cells average 6 to 10 $\times 10^{9}$/litre and platelets 150–400 $\times 10^{9}$/litre. If the laboratory technician had actually to count the cells in a cubic millimetre the task would be Herculean indeed. You might like to calculate how long it would take you to count up to five million, without stopping, at the rate of 20 per second. It works out somewhere near 70 hours. From this it is obvious that a simple method had to be devised for counting cells in blood.

The method involves diluting the blood to a strength of 1 in 200 with a special diluting liquid that will not damage the cells in any way. The red cells present in $\frac{1}{50}$ of a cubic millimetre are counted and the result is multiplied by 50 and 200 to give the number present in 1 cubic millimetre. The figure is correct within 10 000 cells provided the actual counting has been done carefully.

White-cell counts are done in a similar fashion but the blood is first diluted to a strength of 1 in 20. The diluting fluid is of such a nature that the red cells present are destroyed but the white cells are untouched. This makes counting a simpler task. The counting chamber is marked out in large squares for white-cell counts, each large square having an area of 1 square millimetre. The volume of dilute blood appearing over one of these large squares is $1 \times \frac{1}{10}\,\text{mm}^3$. Hence the number of white cells appearing within the boundaries of one large square is the number present in $0.1\,\text{mm}^3$ of blood diluted to a strength of 1 in 20. This number has only to be multiplied by 200 (10 and 20) to give the number of white cells in 1 cubic millimetre of pure blood. For greater accuracy more large squares are used than just one. Four is a convenient number and the cells counted are then multiplied by 50 to give the final figure.

Differentiating between the different types of white cells is a skill that comes only from experience, but what the expert discovers when he looks down his microscope can be turned into percentage figures by anyone who can multiply and divide.

As the numbers of all these cells fluctuate rather widely it is usual to express them in percentage figures of the total number.

URINE

Another source of material for laboratory investigation is urine. Like blood, this is a solution of many substances and the amounts of solutes can be measured. The average composition is: water, 96%; urea, 2%; various salts, chiefly sodium chloride, 2%.

In health the amount of urine excreted varies between 500 and 2000 ml, and the quantity depends on intake, sweating, external temperature and exercise. Increased output occurs whenever the amount of fluid consumed is increased or when there is a drop in the temperature of the environment. In some diseases there is an increase in output, as in diabetes mellitus. In this condition increased quantities of water are needed to excrete the glucose in solution. In the condition called diabetes insipidus there is a large output because antidiuretic hormone production is deficient. This hormone regulates the reabsorption of water in the renal tubules. Shortage of it allows an extra large proportion of the water in the body to be discharged as urine.

Diuretics are drugs which encourage the output of urine. In some conditions where oedema occurs such drugs are used extensively. Some of them, especially the mercurial diuretics, can damage the kidney and must be used with care. Caffeine, which is present in tea and coffee, has a diuretic effect.

The specific gravity of urine is the weight of a certain quantity of urine compared with the weight of an equal volume of water. It reflects the quantity of dissolved matter in the urine; the greater the quantity of solute the higher the specific gravity, and *vice versa*. Specific gravities are usually expressed as a comparison with the weight of 1 ml of water, which is approximately 1 gram; but in urine analysis it is more convenient to use the weight of 1 litre of water, which is about 1000 g. So a specific gravity of urine of 1025 indicates that there are 25 g of solutes in each litre.

It would be possible to find the specific gravity of urine by actually weighing a specimen; but it is far more convenient to use an instrument called a urinometer. This

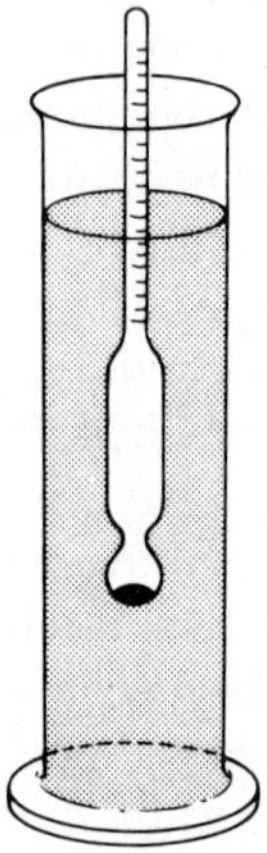

A urinometer

is a special form of hydrometer adapted for use in urine; and the stem is graduated so that specific gravities can be read off directly. The urinometer is immersed in the urine and should not touch the containing vessel at any point. When the urinometer comes to rest the depth to which it has sunk is noted and the figure on the scale which is level with the surface of the urine is the specific gravity of that specimen. Most urinometers are graduated from 0 at the top to 50 at the base of the stem. Whatever figure is read off is added to 1000 to give the final reading.

In health the specific gravity of urine usually varies between 1002 and 1040. As the total amount of waste matter to be excreted in 24 hours is fairly constant in normal healthy people, this variation in specific gravity is caused by the variable amounts of water and other liquids taken. The most concentrated specimen is usually that passed on rising in the morning.

When the kidney is damaged it loses its ability to concentrate urine, and the specific gravity remains constant irrespective of the variations in the amount of fluid consumed. The figure is often constant at about 1010 to 1012. It is easy to see how this happens. A normal healthy kidney can pack all the waste products passing through it into whatever water is available, whereas a diseased kidney cannot do so. If there is only a little water available the diseased kidney will get rid of some of the waste, but any that is left over has to return to the general circulation. If there is plenty of water the diseased kidney is able to excrete its normal quota and is able to get rid of some of the backlog as well. So, no matter what the condition may be, the specific gravity remains the same. Nurses are usually entrusted with the determination of specific gravity and they should make every effort to see that it is done accurately. If there is an insufficient quantity of urine to allow the urinometer to float without touching the bottom of the jar the specific gravity can be measured by adding an identical amount of water and multiplying the reading by 2. This is, however, an extremely inaccurate method and ideally the urine should be sent to the laboratory or specific gravity beads used. These beads can be obtained in sets; each bead is marked with a different specific gravity. Whichever bead will float in the urine denotes the correct reading.

CEREBROSPINAL FLUID

Around the brain and spinal cord in the ventricles of the brain and the central canal of the cord there is a liquid called the cerebrospinal fluid (CSF). Examination of this fluid is an important clinical routine. It is a clear, colourless alkaline fluid with a specific gravity of 1005 to 1008. It contains much the same constituents as plasma, but without the plasma proteins; there are also significant differences in the concentration of the solutes.

There are 125 ml of CSF in the choroid plexuses of the brain ventricles and it is reabsorbed into the capillaries of the arachnoid matter. If CSF is allowed to escape it is reformed at the rate of 500 ml/day.

The pressure that exists in the CSF depends on the position of the body; when lying flat it is sufficient to support 100 to 200 mm of water; in the erect position it is about double this figure. In many conditions, such as head injury, tumour of the brain or meningitis, the pressure is raised and the amounts of solute are altered. Specimens are usually taken by 'lumbar puncture', in which a needle is inserted into the fluid where it extends into a space below the end of the spinal cord.

ELECTROLYTES

Many of the solutes in the various fluids of the body carry an electrical charge. They are electrolytes and contain *ions*, which are atoms that have lost or gained one or two electrons and have therefore become electrically charged. They can also partake in chemical changes.

Their ability to partake in chemical change depends not on their weight but on their electrical charge and so it is preferable to measure their chemical ability rather than their weight.

Until the introduction of S.I. units the unit of chemical combining power was the milliequivalent. Nowadays this is expressed as mmol/litre. The method for converting one to the other is given in Chapter 9. (For Table of Normal Values see the Appendix.)

Electrolytes are of two kinds: those carrying negative charges and those carrying positive charges. Those carrying negative charges are called *anions* and those carrying positive charges are called *cations*. Cations can unite chemically with anions to form whole molecules and herein lies the secret of the balance of electrolytes in the body.

Taken as a whole the healthy body is electrically neutral. In other words such is the chemistry of the body that the number of cations and the number of anions are equal. Local imbalances are bound to occur but are soon corrected to keep the whole system stable. Imbalances probably occur in every disease, and in some diseases on a scale large enough to upset the normal activities of the cells. In some illnesses the imbalance may be so severe that death occurs rapidly and great effort must be made to keep the electrolytes balanced.

In any condition where there is loss of body fluids there will also be loss of electrolytes and consequent upset in the delicate balance. In vomiting, diarrhoea, burns, haemorrhage and shock, gross imbalances are met with and the first consideration of the doctor is to correct them.

This is usually achieved by using intravenous fluids and it is the task of the nurse to ensure that the patient

Table 6. Normal Levels of some Constituents of Body Fluids

Body constituent	*Concentration (mmol/litre)*
Sodium	140
Chloride	100
Potassium	30
Bicarbonate	30

receives the correct amount. When taking responsibility for an infusion, it should be remembered that to give too much or too little can be dangerous for the patient and that complete accuracy is essential. Table 6 gives the levels of those constituents in body fluids which are most frequently assessed.

10 Solutions

A solution occurs when any two substances are mixed together so intimately that their *molecules* are mingled in juxtaposition. Any two substances can form solutions provided that the mixing is on a molecular level, but only certain substances can mix together in this way. The commonest form of solution is that of a solid in a liquid, but soda water is a solution of water and carbon dioxide, i.e. a gas dissolved in a liquid, and many kinds of oil are soluble in alcohol, i.e. one liquid dissolved in another. Gases also may hold substances in solution, e.g. air may take up a certain amount of water and the mixture may be regarded as water dissolved in air.

Metal alloys are solutions of solids, although they are usually mixed while the solids are in a liquid state. This is not always the case, however, and gold and lead laid together in thin sheets and subject to pressure will coalesce to form a metal alloy. Stirring sugar into tea gives us an everyday example of a solution of a solid in a liquid.

In hospitals the word 'solution' usually refers to a liquid, a liquid in which two liquids have been mixed together or one in which a solid has been dissolved in a liquid. The substance dissolved or the lesser quantity is referred to as the *solute*, while the liquid in which the solute has been dissolved is called the *solvent*. Sometimes words other than solvent are used, such as diluent, vehicle or medium. Essentially they mean the same thing.

A good everyday example of a solution used in hospitals is saline. This is merely salty water. Salt is the solute and water is the solvent. Chlorhexidine lotion is a solution of chlorhexidine in water. Chlorhexidine is the solute and water is the solvent. (Spirit is used as the solvent for some purposes.) When one uses ether to remove grease from the skin one is using the solvent powers of ether. Ether is the solvent and the grease is the solute.

Almost always the solutions in hospitals use water as the solvent. When alcohol is used the solution is usually called a tincture. If the solvent is one that evaporates very quickly leaving the solvent behind as a solid the solution may be called a collodion.

The nurse's duties very rarely include the making of solutions other than those with water as the solvent. Preparation of all others is normally undertaken by the pharmacist, who is trained especially for such work. So too with substances for injection. Anything that has to be injected must be prepared under the strictest aseptic precautions and it is better to have a special department with specially trained staff for such work. Although this is so, nurses frequently have to make up solutions such as penicillin, streptomycin, thiopentone and local anaesthetics, so it is necessary for them to know how to make specified strength solutions with a high degree of accuracy. Since this book is concerned merely with mathematics, stress has not been laid on the aseptic precautions that are essential to perfect nursing technique. Hence no such details are included here though a reminder has sometimes been added.

Very many solutions are used in hospitals and it is convenient to separate them under headings and categories.

1. Solutions for external application to the body, such as hexachlorophane, acriflavine, Eusol.
2. Solutions for the disinfection of substances to be used again, such as phenol, Sudol.

3. Solutions for the disinfection of discharges and excreta which will be discarded, such as Sudol.
4. Solutions for the sterilization of instruments, such as glutaraldehyde, formalin and chlorhexidine.
5. Solutions for application to mucous surfaces, such as cocaine, hydrogen peroxide, potassium permanganate, glycerin.
6. Solutions for intramuscular injection, such as morphine, penicillin.

The nurse may be called upon to make up such solutions and she *must* be able to do so accurately. Some solutions are made from drugs of extreme potency; sometimes the solute is in powder or crystal or tablet form; sometimes the solvent is water, but this may have to be distilled water or pyrogen-free sterile water. For external soaks, baths, mouthwashes and disinfectants ordinary tap water is usually suitable. For silver nitrate solutions distilled water is necessary. For all solutions for injection pyrogen-free sterile water is required, together with an aseptic technique.

All this needs an understanding of the terminology and the arithmetic of solutions before a nurse can proceed with confidence. Two abbreviations may cause some confusion at first. They are 'v/v solution' and 'w/v solution'.

v/v solutions are those in which the amount of solute and the amount of the solvent can both be measured in volume units. For instance cetrimide is a liquid and a measure of capacity is used to describe the quantity. Water can be similarly measured so that a solution of Milton can readily be made with millilitre and litre measures.

w/v solutions are those in which the solute is a solid and must be measured in *weight* units. The solvent is measured in *volume* units but for the calculation of the strength the volume units of the solvent are converted into weight units. The strength is then calculated with both substances expressed in *weight* units. Essentially that is all there is to the calculation of w/v solutions and it is no more difficult than the calculation of v/v solution strengths. The relationship between volume and weight in the metric system is helpful as one millilitre of water weighs one gram. A litre of water weighs one kilogram and so on.

Examples

1. Using a millilitre measure pour out 20 ml of red ink. Empty this into a litre measure. Add water to the large measure to make a total of 1 litre. You have now made a v/v solution of red ink. The strength is 20 ml in 1 litre; this is 1 in 50.
2. Add 4 g of salt to 300 ml of water. One millilitre weighs 1 g, therefore 300 ml weighs 300 g. The weight of the solution is 300 g + 4 g = 304 g. 4 g of salt in 304 g = 1 g in 76 g. You have now made a w/v solution.

STRENGTHS OF SOLUTIONS

Ratio strengths

The strength of a solution can be expressed in three ways, ratio strength, percentage strength and dose strength. In the foregoing two exercises ratio strength has been used—one part in so many parts. To find the ratio strength of a solution the *total quantity of the solution* is divided by the *amount of solute* and the answer is expressed as one in whatever the figure may be. Both the quantities must be in the same units to find the strength. It does not matter what units are used provided they are the same for solute and total quantity. Therefore, the rules for finding ratio strength of a solution are thus:

1. Find the quantity of solute.

2. Find the total quantity of solution in the same units.
3. Divide the larger quantity by the smaller.
4. Express the answers as one in this quotient.

Actually the answer can be written down in three ways. It can be written as 'one in something' which is the most expressive way, or in true ratio form with a colon between the two numbers, e.g. 1:20, 1:40, etc., or in simple fractional form, e.g. $\frac{1}{20}$, $\frac{1}{40}$, etc.

Examples

Find the ratio strength of a solution in which 7 ml of pure substance have been added to 203 ml of water.

Quantity of solute = 7 ml
Total quantity of solution = 203 ml of water + 7 ml solute
= 210 ml
210 ÷ 7 = 30
∴ strength is 1 in 30

This strength can also be written 1:30 or $\frac{1}{30}$.

Find the ratio strength when 300 ml is made up to 3 litres with water.

Amount of solute = 300 ml
Total amount of solution = 3 litres
= 3000 ml
3000 ÷ 300 = 10
∴ strength is 1 in 10

This strength can also be written as 1:10 or $\frac{1}{10}$.

Note that in the first example it was necessary to find the total quantity by adding the amount of solute and the amount of solvent, whereas in the second example the wording of the question made it clear that there was a total of 3 litres. All such questions must be read very carefully to make sure whether the quantity of solvent is mentioned or the total quantity of solution.

Ratio strengths are perfect examples of fractions. If you turn back to page 17 you will read that the denominator of a fraction expresses the total number of parts available and that the numerator expresses the number of parts to be considered in any particular instance. Take the ratio strength 1 in 60 as an example. Put into fractional form $\frac{1}{60}$ it tells us that there are 60 parts altogether, the denominator, and that 1 part, the numerator, is pure drug. In all ratio strengths the amount of pure drug is expressed as 1 part while the total quantity varies, 10 parts, 20 parts, 1000 parts, etc.

Percentage strengths

Quite frequently strength is expressed as a percentage instead of a ratio. This has been explained in Chapter 7 but a little application of that chapter is in order in this particular context. To find the percentage strength of a solution divide the amount of solute by the total quantity of solution and multiply by 100. As usual the amounts of solute and solution must be in the same units. Note too that once again the total quantity of solution is required and not merely the amount of solvent.

If the strength of a solution is already expressed in ratio form it can be turned into percentage form by expressing the ratio as a fraction and multiplying it by 100. Conversely, to change percentage strength to ratio strength write down the percentage figure as a fraction (with 100 as the denominator) and divide the denominator by the numerator in the margin. The quotient gives the ratio strength.

Examples

What is the percentage strength when 1 ml of disinfectant concentrate is made up to 80 ml with water?

$$\text{Amount of solute} = 1 \text{ ml}$$
$$\text{Total amount of solution} = 80 \text{ ml}$$
$$\therefore \text{ Percentage strength} = \tfrac{1}{80} \times 100$$
$$= \tfrac{10}{8}$$
$$= 1\tfrac{1}{4}\%$$

What is the percentage strength when 3 g of silver nitrate is dissolved in 200 ml of water (distilled)? (This is a w/v solution so both items must be expressed in weight units.)

$$\text{Amount of solute} = 3 \text{ g}$$
$$\text{Total amount of solution} = 200 \text{ ml}$$
$$200 \text{ ml weighs } 200 \text{ g}$$
$$\therefore \text{ percentage strength} = \frac{3}{200} \times 100$$
$$= \frac{3}{2} \times 1$$
$$= 1\tfrac{1}{2}$$

This is expressed as $1\tfrac{1}{2}\%$ or 1.5%

If you are told that the sodium hypochlorite you are using is 1 in 80, what percentage strength would this be?

$$\text{Ratio strength} = 1 \text{ in } 80$$
$$\therefore \text{ percentage strength} = \tfrac{1}{80} \times 100$$
$$= \tfrac{5}{4}$$
$$= 1\tfrac{1}{4}\%$$

Express 20% as a ratio strength.

$$\text{Percentage strength} = 20$$
$$\therefore \text{ ratio strength } \tfrac{20}{100} = \tfrac{1}{5}$$
$$= 1 \text{ in } 5$$

Dose strength

Stating the strength of a solution in its dose strength is an extremely simple and easy-to-understand method. A certain quantity of drug is dissolved in a certain quantity of solvent and this is stated on the label. Insulin was probably the best example. The strength was stated as so many units per ml. 20, 40 and 80 units per ml were the usual strengths. Many of the antibiotics are similarly expressed in dose strength, penicillin 100 000 units per ml, streptomycin 1 g in 2 ml, and so on.

The usual problem with such drugs is to calculate the amount of solution to be given to ensure a certain quantity of drug. This is very simple arithmetic but accuracy is of vital importance.

Insulin. Insulin is a drug which frequently caused a number of problems to the nurses who had to calculate the dosage. It used to be supplied in strengths of 20, 40 and 80 units per ml. This could be simplified by thinking of 20 units per ml as being single strength. This meant that 40 units per ml was double strength, and 80 units per ml quadruple strength. It is quite easy to see that if a patient required 20 units of insulin one should measure:

1 ml of insulin with 20 units per ml
0.5 ml of insulin with 40 units per ml
0.25 ml of insulin with 80 units per ml

Due to the confusion caused by this system, a single strength of insulin was introduced on 1st March 1983. This contains 100 units per ml. All the other strengths were withdrawn from circulation. At the same time, special syringes were produced. There are two sizes of these. The larger will hold 1 ml or 100 units, the smaller will hold 0.5 ml or 50 units of insulin. It is hoped that this will greatly increase the safety to diabetics who have to use this drug.

It is now worthwhile reading the following examples and then attempting the exercises.

Examples
A diabetic is to receive 20 units of soluble insulin. What quantity will be given from a stock of 40 units per ml?

There are 40 units in 1 ml
$\therefore$ 1 unit in $\frac{1}{40}$ ml
$\therefore$ 20 units in $\frac{1}{40} \times 20$ ml $= \frac{20}{40}$
$= \frac{1}{2}$ ml
$\therefore$ amount to be given is 0.5 ml

How would you give a patient 60 units of insulin from a stock of 80 units per ml?

There are 80 units in 1 ml
$\therefore$ 1 unit in $\frac{1}{80}$ ml
$\therefore$ 60 units in $\frac{1}{80} \times 60$ ml $= \frac{60}{80}$
$\therefore$ you would give 0.75 ml

A patient is to have streptomycin 0.75 g daily. What quantity of solution will be given from a bottle labelled 2 g per ml?

There are 2 g in 1 ml
$\therefore$ 1 g in $\frac{1}{2}$ ml
$\therefore$ $\frac{3}{4}$ g in $\frac{1}{2} \times \frac{3}{4}$ ml $= \frac{3}{8}$ ml
$\therefore$ 0.375 ml will be given each day

How could you give a child 7.5 mg of morphine if the stock bottle is labelled 10 mg in 1 ml?

There are 10 mg in 1 ml
$\therefore$ 1 ml in $\frac{1}{10}$ ml

$$\therefore \frac{1}{10} \times 7\tfrac{1}{2} = \frac{1 \times \overset{3}{\cancel{15}}}{\underset{2}{\cancel{10}} \times 2}$$

$$= \tfrac{3}{4}$$

$$= 0.75$$

∴ you would give the child 0.75 ml

Exercises

1. What quantity is required to give the correct amount of insulin in each of the following?
   (*a*) 32 units from 40 units per ml
   (*b*) 16 units from 20 units per ml
   (*c*) 12 units from 20 units per ml
   (*d*) 60 units from 80 units per ml
   (*e*) 6 units from 20 units per ml
   (*f*) 44 units from 40 units per ml
   (*g*) 15 units from 20 units per ml

2. Calculate the ratio strength of each of the following: (calculate all as if they were v/v solutions, ignoring the fact that some could be more correctly stated as w/v solutions).
   (*a*) Sudol 10 ml added to 390 ml water
   (*b*) 0.2 ml chlorhexidine in 1 litre of solution
   (*c*) 4 ml of cetrimide in 600 ml of solution
   (*d*) 300 mg of cocaine in 60 ml of water
   (*e*) Five litres of solution containing 25 ml of sodium hypochlorite (Milton)
   (*f*) Silver nitrate 120 mg in 30 ml of water

3. Convert each of the following to percentage strengths:
   (*a*) Sodium hypochlorite (Milton) 1 in 80
   (*b*) Chlorhexidine 1 in 1000
   (*c*) Sudol 1 in 40
   (*d*) Cetrimide 1 in 100

4. Convert each of the following to ratio strengths:
   (*a*) Sodium citrate $2\frac{1}{2}$%

(*b*) Magnesium sulphate 3%
(*c*) Cocaine 4%
(*d*) Sodium bicarbonate 1%
(*e*) Dextrose 5%

5. Complete the blank spaces in the following chart:

Amount of pure drug	*Total amount of solution*	*Ratio strength*	*Percentage strength*
(*a*)	100 ml		2%
(*b*)	2 pints	1 in 10	
(*c*) 3 ml			1%
(*d*) 15 ml		1 in 80	
(*e*) 4 ml			5/8%
(*f*) 0.25 ml		1 in 1000	
(*g*)	30 litres		0.01%
(*h*)	40 ml		20%
(*i*)	120 ml		2½%
(*j*)	2 litres		½%
(*k*)	1½ pints	1 in 60	
(*l*)	500 ml		0.2%
(*m*) 4 ml			1¼%
(*n*) 0.5 ml		1 in 80	

6. List three solutions used in your hospital for each of the following tasks. Give the ratio strength and the percentage strength. Work out how much pure drug you would need to make various appropriate quantities.
(*a*) Solutions used for the sterilization of surgical instruments.
(*b*) Solutions used for mouthwashes, rectal washout, gargles, etc.
(*c*) Solutions for irrigation of the stomach.

(*d*) Solutions used for bladder washout.
(*e*) Solutions used for irrigation of wounds.
(*f*) Solutions used for eye drops.

11 Calculation of Drug Dosages and Dilution of Lotions

A nurse is often required to give a certain strength of drug or to use a certain strength of lotion, and all she or he has is something stronger. The nurse has the right substance but it is too strong. We can all think of instances when such has been the case. We want to give morphine 15 mg and have only 20 mg, or we wish to use chlorhexidine 1 in 5000 when we are supplied with strength 1 in 1000.

Such problems are constantly arising and if the nurse cannot work out exactly how the dilution is to be performed, there is a risk that she or he will be tempted to go by guesswork. Getting it 'somewhere near' may be of little consequence when the dilution is required for the sterilization of contaminated items, but there is no room for guesswork where drugs are concerned, particularly when the drug is a dangerous one. We must be exact or else own up to our ignorance and hand over to someone who knows better. There is no disgrace in doing so, whereas proceeding in ignorance is criminal folly, and may cost a life.

When one follows the working of a few examples it is surprising how simple the process is. But one *must* follow thc reasoning and work out plenty of theoretical examples so that when the situation arises in real life one can say to oneself, 'Ah! This is something I have mastered. I am on sure ground here', and can proceed with calm assurance.

Sometimes the problem is so simple that one can do the arithmetic mentally. As a general rule, however, it is better to take pencil and paper to make absolutely sure that there is no error.

For instance, in an example such as, 'How would you give morphine 7.5 mg if you have only ampoules of 15 mg?' it is obvious that 7.5 is half of 15 and that one should halve the liquid and discard the remainder. But if asked to give 6 mg when only ampoules of 20 mg are available, the answer may not be so obvious. We require some simple rule of thumb that will apply to all cases.

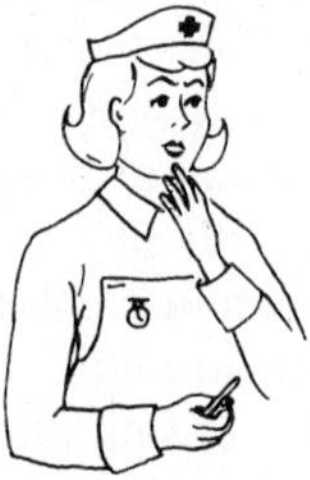

? 6 from 20

There is such a rule and stripped to its bare bones it states: *Divide the strength you want by the strength you have*.

This should be memorized so that you can wake up in bed at three o'clock in the morning and repeat it without any doubt in your mind whatsoever.

Say to yourself whenever you have to deal with any of these problems, 'What strength do I *want*?' Write it down as a fraction.

Next you say to yourself, 'What strength have I *got*?' Write this alongside as another fraction and insert a division sign between the two.

From here on it is simple arithmetic. We have two fractions the first of which is going to be divided by the second. You will remember that the way to divide by a fraction is to turn it upside down and multiply by it. There will usually be some cancelling to do and the end result will be a fraction. This fraction is what you are after as it tells you how much of the substance you will need to take from the stock. For instance, if the resulting fraction is $\frac{1}{10}$ you will need to take $\frac{1}{10}$ of the final quantity from the stock and add to it sufficient water from the tap or from a bottle of sterile water to make it up to the quantity required.

Let us apply the rules to the first easy example that we mentioned before, that of giving 7.5 mg of morphine when only 15 mg ampoules are available. We already know the answer, so if our arithmetic comes out to anything different we had better examine the arithmetic.

The rule is—divide the strength you want by the strength you have.

$$\begin{aligned} \text{Strength wanted} &= 7.5 \text{ mg} \\ \text{Strength you have} &= 15 \text{ mg in } 1 \text{ ml} \\ 7\tfrac{1}{2} \div 15 &= \tfrac{15}{2} \div \tfrac{15}{1} \\ &= \tfrac{15}{2} \times \tfrac{1}{15} \\ &= \tfrac{1}{2} \end{aligned}$$

Therefore half the quantity in the 15 mg ampoule will contain 7.5 mg. The other half is discarded.

Now let us have a look at the second example quoted. It said—how would you give 6 mg if you had only 20 mg ampoules.

Go about it in exactly the same way.

$$\begin{aligned} \text{Strength wanted} &= 6 \text{ mg} \\ \text{Strength supplied} &= 20 \text{ mg in } 1 \text{ ml} \\ 6 \div 20 &= \frac{6}{20} \\ &= \frac{\overset{3}{\cancel{6}}}{\underset{10}{\cancel{20}}} \\ &= \tfrac{3}{10} \end{aligned}$$

Therefore three-tenths of 1 ml will contain 6 mg. The remaining seven-tenths are discarded.

In some instances the amounts to be dealt with are very small quantities. The rule applies equally well.

How can 400 micrograms (μg) of Digoxin be given if the ward stock carries only ampoules of 600 μg of Digoxin?

Strength wanted= 400 μg

Strength supplied= 600 μg in 1 ml

$$400 \div 600 = \frac{400}{600}$$

Therefore $\frac{2}{3}$ ml contains the required dose; the remaining $\frac{1}{3}$ is discarded.

Here is another example with lotions. How would you prepare from a stock bottle of chlorhexidine of strength 1 in 500, a litre of lotion of strength 1 in 2500?

Strength wanted = 1/2500

Stock strength = 1/500

$$\frac{1}{2500} \div \frac{1}{500} = \frac{1}{2500} \times \frac{500}{1}$$
$$= \frac{5}{25}$$
$$= \frac{1}{5}$$

Therefore $\frac{1}{5}$ of 1 litre is taken from the stock bottle—that is $\frac{1}{5}$ of 1000 ml = 200 ml, and the litre is made up by adding tap water.

When dealing with percentage solutions, the task becomes extremely simple because fractions need not enter into the calculation at all. The rule of dividing the strength required by the strength you have still holds.

For instance—How much chloroxylenol 10% is required to make 1 litre of 1% solution?

Strength wanted= 1%

Strength of stock= 10%

$$1 \div 10 = \frac{1}{10}$$

Therefore you will need $\frac{1}{10}$ of 1 litre from the 10% bottle, which is 100 ml.

CHILDREN'S DOSAGES

The doses of drugs given in pharmacopoeias are usually adult doses. Special doses are given for children. Many methods have been used in the past to calculate children's dosages. Nowadays, however, it is generally accepted that the most accurate way in which to do this is to base the dosage on the body surface area of the child. Catzel* produced a formula by which the surface area can be calculated from the height and the weight of the child. The figure is then expressed as a percentage of the surface area of the average adult, and the dosage for the child is that percentage of the dosage for an adult. It is usually the nurse who has to record these heights and weights and it is a considerable responsibility for her to have to undertake since a mistake may cause the doctor to write an incorrect prescription and the child to receive a dosage which will be too great. This means that all nurses, however senior, should have all heights and weights checked by a second person.

Nurses do not usually have to prescribe drugs, but they do have to measure and administer them. When measuring children's doses it is sometimes necessary to calculate quite small amounts from a stock solution which has been prepared for adults. Below are given a few doses to calculate, which can be worked out quite easily if the formula given earlier in the chapter is used. Maybe if it is written again as a calculation it will assist you:

$$\frac{\text{Strength you want}}{\text{Strength you have}} = \text{Amount}$$

Therefore if a child requires 125 mg of i.m. ampicillin, and

*CATZEL, P. (1966) *Paediatric Prescriber*, 3rd ed. Oxford: Blackwell Scientific.

the stock solution is 250 mg in 2 ml, the dose is calculated in the following way

Strength you want = 125 mg
Strength you have = 250 mg in 2 ml

$$125 \div \frac{250}{2} = \frac{125 \times 2}{250}$$
$$= 1 \text{ ml}$$

Therefore the child requires 1 ml of the solution.

Now try a few more:

Dose required		*Stock solution*
1. Oral ampicillin	62.5 mg	125 mg/5 ml
2. Soluble aspirin	75 mg	300 mg tablet
3. Chloral hydrate	500 mg	100 mg/1 ml
4. Chloral hydrate	1 gram	100 mg/1 ml
5. Elixir Digoxin	0.01 mg	0.05 mg/1 ml
6. Elixir Digoxin	0.03 mg	0.05 mg/1 ml
7. Elixir Digoxin	0.08 mg	0.05 mg/1 ml
8. Phenergan elixir	8 mg	5 mg/5 ml

Exercises

1. How would you give a patient an injection of Omnopon 15 mg from an ampoule marked 20 mg?

2. How much potassium permanganate solution 50% is required to prepare a general bath containing 90 litres of 2% strength?

3. Sodium hypochlorite 5% is supplied to the ward. How much will be required to make 2.5 litres 1 in 80 for babies' bottles?

4. How much silver nitrate solution strength 1 in 1000 must be used to prepare 1200 ml of solution strength 1 in 3000 for irrigation of the bladder? How much distilled water should be added?

5. An insulin bottle is marked 40 units per ml. How much will contain 25 units?

6. A bottle of morphine sulphate solution is labelled 15 mg in 2 ml. How much must be drawn up if it is required to give 10 mg?
7. An ampoule of solution is marked Pethidine Hyd. 100 mg, Promethazine Hyd. 50 mg in 2 ml. If 1.5 ml are injected how much pethidine and how much promethazine have been administered?
8. How much sudol 1 in 20 is required to make a litre of 1 in 160?
9. How would you prepare 600 ml of chlorhexidine of strength 1 in 1500 from a stock of 1 in 1000?
10. How much magnesium sulphate solution 1 in 5 is needed to make 300 ml of 1 in 20?
11. How much 1 in 2000 solution is needed to make 200 ml of 1 in 5000?
12. If 60 mg of morphine is dissolved in 4 ml of water, how much contains 20 mg?
13. How much water must be added to 300 ml of 20% strength glucose to make it 5%?
14. Prepare 200 ml of cetrimide 0.1% solution from stock of 1%.
15. How much 20% alcohol solution can be made from 1 litre of 95%.
16. Prepare 1000 ml of 1 in 8000 potassium permanganate solution from 0.1% stock.
17. Make 250 ml cocaine solution 1% from 2%.

12 Thermometry

Quite early in man's search for knowledge it was realized that an accurate instrument for measuring temperature changes was required. Answers to questions such as, 'How much hotter or colder is this substance now that I have experimented with it?' or 'Is today's temperature more or less than yesterday's?' needed urgent answers in precise terms before real advances could take place.

Much of the early work done on temperature was done by men who were seeking to enhance their country's sea power. It was beginning to be realized that wind strengths and changes were connected with temperature in adjoining areas, and as ships were dependent entirely on the winds, there would be definite advantages to the navies that could predict how the wind was going to blow, just as present-day meteorologists supply the information on which our air fleets rely. Without thermometers, a serious gap is left.

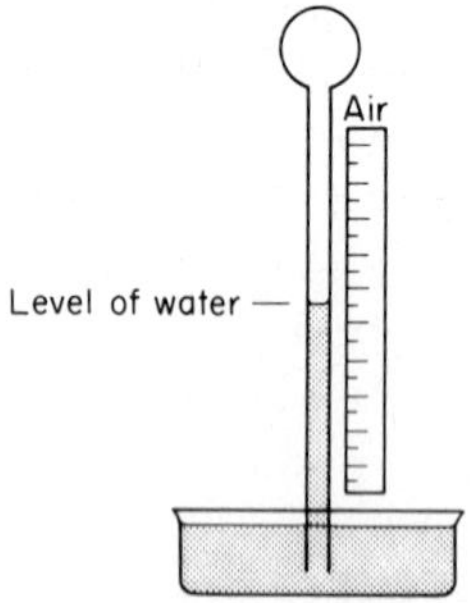

Galileo's thermometer

Galileo, the sixteenth-century genius, invented among all his other wonderful creations a kind of thermometer. This he did in 1593 and it is surprising that such a simple instrument was not invented before. It is something that any nurse could set up for herself. It consists of a flask with a cork in its neck through which passes a glass tube. This is turned upside down with the end of the tube under the surface of some water in a glass. The air in the glass bulb is heated thus causing it to expand and some of it will bubble away from the end of the tubing. When the air is allowed to cool some water is drawn up into the tubing. The level of the water in the tube will then rise and fall with even slight changes in room temperature. With an ordinary wall thermometer used as a guide it is possible to graduate the tubing quite accurately.

In spite of the extreme sensitivity of this thermometer it has certain drawbacks that make it unsuitable for general use. For one thing, it is bulky and easily broken; variations in atmospheric pressure will also cause the water to rise and fall in the tube independently of temperature; a very long tube indeed would be required for large temperature ranges. It was not long before better thermometers were invented.

Rey, a French doctor, in 1632, used a small bulb and tube filled with water with the end of the tube sealed, similar to our mercury-filled thermometers, but larger. The water expanded along the tube when the bulb was warmed. He used it to detect rises in body temperature and to him can go the honour of inventing the first 'clinical thermometer'. This was quite useless to the climatologists, however. The water froze at low temperatures and between 4°C and 0°C showed an apparent rise in temperature owing to the peculiar property that water has of expanding instead of contracting between those temperatures.

The Florentine Academy took the next steps leading up to 'modern' thermometry. They established the principle that it was necessary to have two easily determined temperatures, one high and one low, that were constant. Any thermometer could then be graduated so that 10 degrees meant the same on one as it meant on any other. These two 'fixed points' would have to be the temperatures of easily available things and were chosen as the temperature of snow or ice during the severest frost of the winter and the rectal temperature of cows or deer. The space in between these two points was then divided into 40 or 80 equal divisions or degrees. The winter temperatures of Florence must have been remarkably constant as several of these Florentine thermometers came to light recently and all showed the temperature of melting ice to be at $13\frac{1}{2}$ degrees. Nowadays we recognize that these temperatures are far too variable to be of practical use for the accuracy that we demand, but at that time the principle constituted a remarkable advance.

The second achievement was the substitution of alcohol for water as the expanding fluid. Alcohol was unfreezable at that time so that comparatively low temperatures could then be recorded. In addition, alcohol expands at a constant rate throughout the whole range of temperatures. Its greatest drawback was that it has a boiling point slightly lower than that of water and could not be used for higher temperatures.

Mercury was first used by a Parisian astronomer, Boulliau, in 1659, and there the matter stood for nearly 50 years until Fahrenheit invented his thermometer in 1712.

Fahrenheit took a small glass bulb with a narrow glass tube leading from it and filled the bulb with mercury. He then heated the mercury until it expanded to fill the tube completely. The end of the tube was then sealed in a flame, and as the mercury cooled it shrank back into the bulb leaving a vacuum behind it. This is the type of thermometer we are familar with today. His next step was to establish two fixed points on the stem of the thermometer. For his lower fixed point he put his thermometer into a mixture of ammoniated salt and ice believing this to be the coldest temperature possible to attain. This was marked zero. His upper fixed point was obtained by placing the thermometer in boiling water. The level to which the mercury rose was marked on the stem and this was labelled 212 degrees. Why Fahrenheit chose these particular figures will probably forever remain a mystery. On this scale the temperature of melting ice is 32 degrees and, as this temperature is the one used to determine the lower fixed points in the two other major scales, it is of far more importance than Fahrenheit's zero. This should be remembered as it is of some importance when the question of conversion from one scale to another is to be considered.

In 1742, Celsius, a Swede working in Switzerland, introduced what has been known as the Centigrade scale.

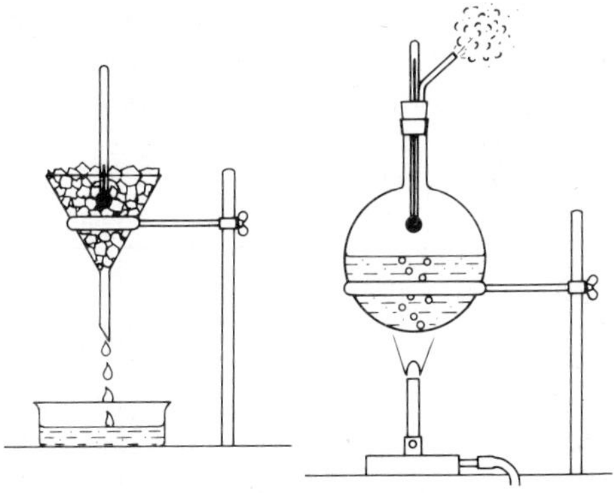

Lower 'fixed point' (32°) from melting ice

Upper 'fixed point' from boiling water

Fahrenheit's thermometer

He used the temperatures of freezing and boiling water as his lower and upper fixed points. The distance between these two points he divided into 100 equal divisions or degrees. At first he called the upper one 0 degrees and the lower one 100 degrees, but 9 years later these were reversed by a fellow worker and were named as we know them today with the freezing point of water at 0 degrees and the boiling point of water at 100 degrees.

The term Centigrade is used in some other countries to denote fractions of a right angle. Therefore when agreement was reached on the International System of Units it was decided that the name 'degree Centigrade' be replaced by the name 'degree Celsius'.

CONVERSION FROM ONE SCALE TO ANOTHER

Until recently the Fahrenheit scale was used extensively in Great Britain and it is the scale that still conveys most meaning to many nurses. When one hears that the temperature on a certain day was 90°F in the shade, a picture of oppressive heat is conjured up in one's mind. But if one hears that the temperature was 32.2°C in the shade, it conveys very little impression unless one has

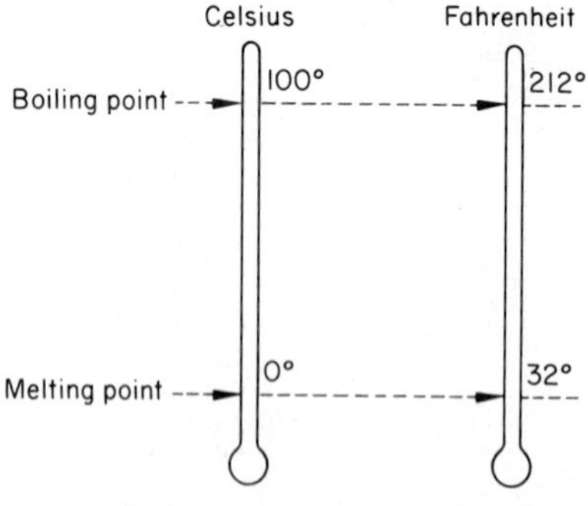

Equivalent points on the two scales

become used to dealing with the Celsius scale, and then one realizes that it is the same thing. It is a question of familiarity. Until such familiarity has been cultivated it is necessary to be able to convert from one scale to the other.

There are two methods for conversion, both of which we shall consider.

Method 1

The rules for conversion are very simple. Let us write them down and then examine them to see how they are derived.

1. To convert degrees Celsius to degrees Fahrenheit multiply the degrees Celsius by $\frac{9}{5}$ and then add 32.
2. To convert degrees Fahrenheit to degrees Celsius, subtract 32 from the degrees Fahrenheit and then multiply by $\frac{5}{9}$.

The usual difficulty that nurses encounter is to remember whether to multiply by $\frac{5}{9}$ or $\frac{9}{5}$. As this can be worked out from first principles in a few moments it need not constitute a major problem. Both scales use the same fixed points, the freezing and boiling points of water. Therefore 0°C and 32°F are equal. So too are 100°C and 212°F. Between 0 and 100 there are obviously 100 divisions, and between 32 and 212 there are 180 divisions. Hence 100 Celsius degrees covers the same range as 180 Fahrenheit degrees. If 100 Celsius divisions is equal to 180 Fahrenheit divisions, 1 Celsius degree must equal 180 divided by 100 Fahrenheit degrees. By simplification, $\frac{180}{100}$ becomes $\frac{9}{5}$. Why this should present any difficulty is hard to see. If a person were to say, 'Here are 100 counters made of black plastic. They have the same value as 180 red beads', anyone could answer the question 'How much is one black counter worth?' This leads logically to the answers to, 'How much are 10, 15 or 75 counters worth?'

The same applies to degrees. If 1°C = $\frac{9}{5}$°F, 10°C = $\frac{9}{5} \times$ 10°F, 20°C = $\frac{9}{5} \times$ 20°F, 75°C = $\frac{9}{5} \times$ 75°F, and so on.

To each of these answers must be added 32. This is because the starting point of both scales is the freezing point of water which is called zero on the Celsius scale but is called 32 on the Fahrenheit scale. In other words, the Fahrenheit scale has got a 'start' on the Celsius; and its 'handicap' must be added after the multiplication if the comparison is going to be 'fair'.

Converting from Fahrenheit to Celsius is carried out by reversing the process. The 'handicap' must be removed first of all so we start by subtracting 32. The next step is to multiply the remainder by $\frac{5}{9}$. This figure is derived in the following way. If 180 Fahrenheit degrees are equal to 100 Celsius degrees, one Fahrenheit degree equals 100 divided by 180 Celsius degrees, $\frac{100}{180} = \frac{5}{9}$ when the simplification has been completed. Hence, if 1 Fahrenheit degree equals $\frac{5}{9}$ of a Celsius degree, 10 Fahrenheit degrees equals $10 \times \frac{5}{9}$ Celsius degrees, and so on.

Examples

Convert 98.6°F to the Celsius scale.

(*a*) Subtract 32:

$$98.6 - 32 = 66.6$$

(*b*) Multiply by $\frac{5}{9}$:

$$\overset{7.4}{\cancel{66.6}} \times \frac{5}{\underset{1}{\cancel{9}}} = 7.4 \times \frac{5}{1}$$

$$= 37$$

$$\therefore 98.6°\text{F} = 37°\text{C}$$

Convert 59°F to the Celsius scale.

(*a*) $$59 - 32 = 27$$

(*b*) $$\overset{3}{\cancel{27}} \times \frac{5}{\underset{1}{\cancel{9}}} = 15$$

$$\therefore 59°\text{F} = 15°\text{C}$$

Convert 12.2°F to the Celsius scale.

(*a*) $$12.2 - 32 = \text{minus } 19.8$$

(*b*) $$\text{minus } \overset{2.2}{\cancel{19.8}} \times \frac{5}{\underset{1}{\cancel{9}}} = \text{minus } 11$$

$$\therefore 12.2°\text{F} = \text{minus } 11°\text{C}$$

Now in the reverse direction:

Convert 10°C to the Fahrenheit scale.

(*a*) Multiply by $\frac{9}{5}$:

$$\overset{2}{\cancel{10}} \times \frac{9}{\underset{1}{\cancel{5}}} = 18$$

(*b*) Add 32:

$$18 + 32 = 50$$

$$\therefore 10°\text{C} = 50°\text{F}$$

Convert 95°C to the Fahrenheit scale.

(*a*) $$\overset{19}{\cancel{95}} \times \frac{9}{\underset{1}{\cancel{5}}} = 171$$

(*b*) $$171 + 32 = 203$$

$$\therefore 95°\text{C} = 203°\text{F}$$

Convert minus 5°C to the Fahrenheit scale.

(*a*) minus $5 \times \frac{9}{5}$ = minus 9
(*b*) minus 9 + 32 = 23
$\therefore$ minus 5°C = 23°F

Method 2

This method may be found by some people to be easier to remember than the first. The steps are as follows:

1st step	add 40
2nd step	(*a*) Multiply by $\frac{5}{9}$ to convert from the Fahrenheit scale to the Celsius scale. or (*b*) Multiply by $\frac{9}{5}$ to convert from the Celsius scale to the Fahrenheit scale.
3rd step	Now the 1st step is reversed, that is, 40 is deducted from the total.

To allow this method to be compared with the first method let us try it on the problems already worked.

Examples

Convert 98.6°F to the Celsius scale.

(*a*) Add 40:

$$98.6 + 40 = 138.6$$

(*b*) Multiply by $\frac{5}{9}$:

$$\frac{\overset{15.4}{\cancel{138.6}} \times 5}{\underset{1}{\cancel{9}}} = 77.0$$

(*c*) Subtract 40:

$$77 - 40 = 37°C$$

Convert 59°C to the Celsius scale.

(*a*) Add 40:

$$59 + 40 = 99$$

(*b*) Multiply by $\frac{5}{9}$:

$$\frac{\overset{11}{\cancel{99}} \times 5}{\underset{1}{\cancel{9}}} = 55$$

(*c*) Subtract 40:

$$55 - 40 = 15°\text{C}$$

Convert 12.2°F to the Celsius scale.

(*a*) Add 40:

$$12.2 + 40 = 52.2$$

(*b*) Multiply by $\frac{5}{9}$:

$$\frac{\overset{5.8}{\cancel{52.2}} \times 5}{\underset{1}{\cancel{9}}} = 29.0$$

(*c*) Subtract 40:

$$29 - 40 = -11°\text{C}$$

Next we shall work in the reverse direction again.

Convert 10°C to the Fahrenheit scale.

(*a*) Add 40:

$$10 + 40 = 50$$

(*b*) Multiply by $\frac{9}{5}$:

$$\frac{\overset{10}{\cancel{50}} \times 9}{\underset{1}{\cancel{5}}} = 90$$

(*c*) Subtract 40:

$$90 - 40 = 50°\text{F}$$

Convert 95°C to the Fahrenheit scale.

(*a*) Add 40:

$$95 + 40 = 135$$

(*b*) Multiply by $\frac{9}{5}$:

$$\frac{\overset{27}{\cancel{135}} \times 9}{\underset{1}{\cancel{5}}} = 243$$

(*c*) Subtract 40:

$$243 - 40 = 203°\text{F}$$

Convert minus 5°C to the Fahrenheit scale.

(*a*) Add 40:

$$-5 + 40 = 35$$

(*b*) Multiply by $\frac{9}{5}$:

$$\frac{\overset{7}{\cancel{35}} \times 9}{\underset{1}{\cancel{5}}} = 63$$

(*c*) Subtract 40:

$$63 - 40 = 23°\text{F}$$

Exercises

1. Give four reasons why mercury is a better liquid to use in themometers than water.

2. What disadvantages are there to water as a thermometer liquid? Are there any advantages?

3. Convert each of the following to the Fahrenheit scale:
(*a*) 3°C (*b*) 18°C (*c*) 25.5°C (*d*) 100°C
(*e*) 36°C (*f*) 42°C (*g*) 50°C (*h*) 70°C

4. Convert each of the following to the Celsius scale:
(*a*) 41°F (*b*) 77°F (*c*) 55.4°F (*d*) 104°F
(*e*) 86°F (*f*) 78.8°F (*g*) 365.9°F (*h*) 212°F

5. State which of the following are true and which false:
(*a*) 0°C = 0°F (*b*) 32°F = 0°C
(*c*) 98.6°F = 37°C (*d*) minus 40°C = minus 4°F
(*e*) 40°F = 40°C (*f*) 100°F = 100°C
(*g*) 92°F = 60°C

THE CLINICAL THERMOMETER

It is possible to take a person's temperature with an ordinary thermometer, especially if it is used rectally, but it is not an easy matter. The glass is usually so thick that the thermometer has to be left in contact with the tissues for a considerable length of time. The bore of the tube is comparatively large compared with that of a clinical thermometer and consequently requires more heat to cause the mercury to expand. The heat lost from the stem of the thermometer may equal that gained from the body if the stem is very long, so the mercury will never be able to climb to a true reading. There is no provision made to prevent the mercury contracting back into the bulb when it is removed from the tissues so that it would have to be read *in situ*.

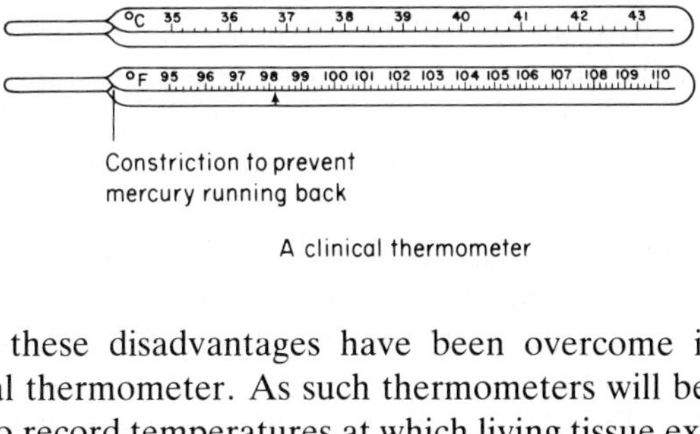

A clinical thermometer

All these disadvantages have been overcome in the clinical thermometer. As such thermometers will be used only to record temperatures at which living tissue exists, it would be pointless to make them so that they are capable of registering the freezing point or the boiling point of water. It is generally considered that animal tissues will die if they are kept at temperatures much below 35°C or over 43.3°C for more than a very short time. Hence a standard clinical thermometer need only register between these limits. Special thermometers are used for recording the sub-normal temperatures of some elderly people and of patients undergoing operations involving hypothermic techniques.

Secondly, to use glass as thick as that used in other types of thermometers is likely to cause considerable delay in the registering of the temperature. This is time that can be ill afforded in the running of a busy ward. Therefore the glass of clinical thermometers is quite thin, particularly round the bulb.

Thirdly, there is need for great accuracy, far more so than is the case with the temperature of a room or boiler where accuracy to one degree is quite sufficient. This accuracy can be attained by making the bore of the thermometer very fine so that the mercury travels further along the stem as it expands. This allows for graduations of one-fifth of a degree or less.

Fourthly, the mercury having expanded, it must be prevented from returning into the bulb as it cools after removal from the body. This is achieved by making the bore of the stem even smaller at a point just above the bulb. Obviously it must not be made so narrow that the mercury cannot be forced back into the bulb, and every nurse soon learns the knack of 'shaking down' the thermometer with a flick of the wrist. Some thermometers are easier to 'shake down' than others, indicating that the size of the constriction varies from one thermometer to another.

Many clinical thermometers have a triangular cross section so that the mercury may be seen more easily. The effect of this peculiar cross-section is to magnify the fine hair-like thread of mercury. Sometimes the glass behind the thread of mercury is coloured, usually white, but sometimes red or blue. The silvery colour stands out more clearly than if the glass behind were transparent.

Most clinical thermometers have the time that it takes to record engraved into the glass at the back. Some are

3-minute thermometers, some 2-minute, some 1- or $\frac{1}{2}$- or even $\frac{1}{4}$-minute. If a 3-minute one is compared with a $\frac{1}{2}$-minute one, it becomes obvious immediately that much of the thickness of the glass has been sacrificed for the sake of recording. You can have a comparatively strong one that takes a much longer time to record or you can have a fragile one that records quickly. Even so, many nurses find that the time recorded on the back is quite unreliable even with an expensive thermometer, and usually they prefer to take no chances and keep the thermometer in position for a full 3 minutes in spite of what is stated on the back.

Conversion tables for transposing Fahrenheit and Celsius

To use Table 7 for conversion from Celsius to Fahrenheit split the temperature into tens, units and decimals and look up the figures for each. Write these down under each other and then add them to find the temperature in

Table 7. To Convert Celsius to Fahrenheit

°C	°F	°C	°F	°C	°F
0	32	1	1.8	0.1	0.18
10	50	2	3.6	0.2	0.36
20	68	3	5.4	0.3	0.54
30	86	4	7.2	0.4	0.72
40	104	5	9.0	0.5	0.9
50	122	6	10.8	0.6	1.08
60	140	7	12.6	0.7	1.26
70	158	8	14.4	0.8	1.44
80	176	9	16.2	0.9	1.62
90	194				
100	212				

degrees Fahrenheit. For example, to convert 48.6°C look up the figures for 40°, then 8° and lastly 0.6°. Enter them thus:

$$\begin{array}{r} 104 \\ 14.4 \\ 1.08 \\ \hline 119.48 \\ \hline \end{array}$$

$$\therefore 48.6°C = 119.48°F$$

The table can be used for temperatures higher than 109.9°C but, as the first column of Fahrenheit degrees has

Table 8. To Convert Fahrenheit to Celsius

°F	°C	°F	°C	°F	°C
30	–1.1	1	0.56	0.1	0.06
40	4.4	2	1.11	0.2	0.11
50	10.0	3	1.67	0.3	0.17
60	15.6	4	2.22	0.4	0.22
70	21.1	5	2.78	0.5	0.28
80	26.7	6	3.33	0.6	0.33
90	32.2	7	3.89	0.7	0.39
100	37.8	8	4.44	0.8	0.44
110	43.3	9	5.0	0.9	0.5
120	48.9				
130	54.4				
140	60.0				
150	65.6				
160	71.1				
170	76.7				
180	82.2				
190	87.8				
200	93.3				
210	98.9				

already had 32 added to make up for the difference between the zero points in the two scales, care must be taken to subtract 32 when looking up the converted figure for the 'tens'. For instance, to find the equivalent of 160°C look up the figure for 100°, then the figure for 60°. Now 32 has been added to both of these figures already, so one lot of 32 must be taken off again to give the final figure. Hence, 100°C = 212°F, 60°C = 140°F and 160°C = 212 + 140 − 32 = 320°F.

Table 8 is for conversion from Fahrenheit to Celsius and is used in the same way. Here again temperatures higher than 219.9°F can be converted with a similar proviso, and that is that the amount of 17.8 must be added to the figure found for anything in the 'tens'. For example 280°F is first split into 200 and 80. 200°F = 93.3°C, 80°F = 26.7°C, therefore 280°F = 93.3 + 26.7 + 17.8 = 137.8°C.

13 Heat and Energy

Temperature is a measurement that tells us the degree of hotness or coldness of a substance. It tells us whether something is hotter or cooler than another object without giving us the slightest indication as to how much *heat* that particular object contains. A good analogy can be made between the quality of wetness in liquids. We can say that rainwater is wetter than sea water, or that normal saline is wetter than Epsom salts solution, just as we can say that such and such an object is hotter than another. To say that one liquid is wetter than another gives us no clue to the quantity of water, just as the temperature gives us no clue to the amount of heat.

It is possible to have a kettle of water containing 1 litre and another containing 4 litres, both having exactly the same temperature, but there will be four times as much *heat* in the 4 litres as there is in the 1 litre. Putting this another way round makes it self-evident. In order to boil both these kettles it will take four times as long to boil the 4 litres as it will to boil the other, provided the size of the gas jet remains the same for both. In other words, one has to put four times as much heat into the large quantity as into the small quantity.

One can think of many examples to illustrate this point. For instance, which would you rather take to bed on a cold night, a hot-water bottle with a 2 litre capacity or a baby's hot water-bottle containing $\frac{1}{4}$ of a litre? Your answer will be that you would prefer the larger one. Why? Because the larger one stays hot longer. It contains more heat than the smaller one and it takes longer for the heat to dissipate. Or again, if you had to iron sheets with an old-fashioned flat iron, would you choose a large one or a small one? A large one because, even though they are heated to the same temperature in the first place, the large one will absorb more heat and will stay hot longer in consequence.

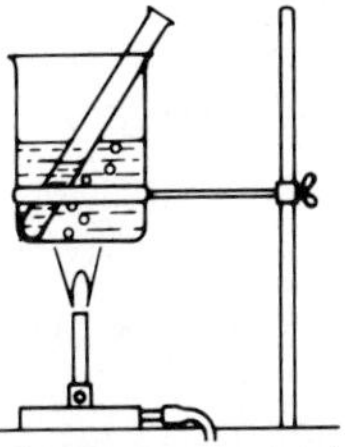

5 ml of water in a test tube
standing in
50 ml of boiling water

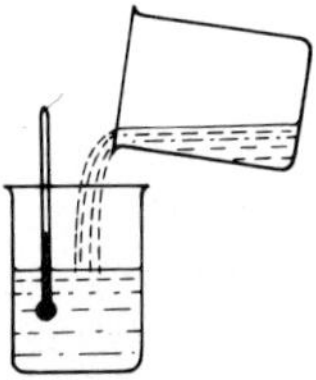

50 ml of boiling water
added to
50 ml of cold water

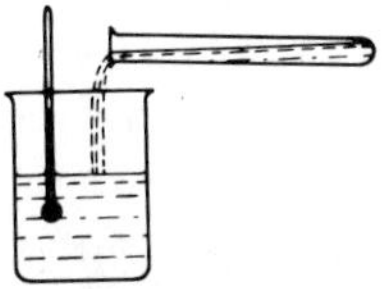

5 ml of boiling water
added to
50 ml of cold water

A simple experiment can be performed to show that different quantities of water at the same temperature contain different quantities of heat in proportion to their volume. Take a beaker of water containing 50 ml and stand a test tube in it containing 5 ml of water. Heat the beaker over a jet. Take the temperature of the water in the beaker and that in the test tube. They should be the same. now take two more beakers of the same size each containing 50 ml of tap water. Take the temperature of this water. Into one pour the water from the heated beaker and into the other pour the water from the test tube. Now take the temperatures of the mixtures. What is the *increase* in temperature in each case? It will be seen that the larger quantity of hot water has increased the temperature of the cold water by ten times the amount achieved by the small quantity, which indicates that the larger quantity contained ten times as much heat as the smaller quantity even though they were heated to the same temperature.

UNITS OF HEAT

Now that it is clear that temperature is not the same as the quantity of heat it can be seen that it has been necessary to invent units that will measure quantities of heat. As in all other cases of measurement a unit or standard is required for purposes of comparison.

The unit quantity of heat is called a *calorie* and is defined as *the quantity of heat that will raise the temperature of one gram of water by one degree Celsius.*

The quantity of heat that is required to raise the temperature of 2 g of water by 1°C is therefore 2 calories. Similarly if 6 g of water is heated sufficiently to raise its temperature by 1°C it will have taken up 6 calories. If 10 g are raised 12°C it will have received $10 \times 12 = 120$ calories, the number of calories being equal to the weight of water in grams multiplied by the rise in temperature by degrees Celsius.

There is also a unit in the British measurements called a British Thermal Unit, or B.T.U. for short. This is defined as the amount of heat required to raise the temperature of 1 lb of water through 1°F. This is equivalent to 252 calories. Calories and British Thermal Units are rather small quantities when it comes to measuring the heat value of gas supplies or food substances, and for these purposes larger units have been devised. Dietetic Calories are equivalent to 1000 of the calories that are written about here. We shall come across dietetic Calories later in this chapter. The heating power of gas is measured in therms, one of which is equivalent to 100 000 B.T.U. How the supply of gas can be adjusted to the demand for it may be illustrated by an example. An iron kettle weighs 3 lb and the water in it weighs 5 lb. Taking the specific heat of iron as $\frac{1}{9}$, the 3 lb kettle is equivalent to $3 \times \frac{1}{9}$ lb of water which equals $\frac{1}{3}$ lb. Hence the weight of the kettle plus the water is equivalent to $5\frac{1}{3}$ lb of water. Therefore it will take $5\frac{1}{3}$ B.T.U. to raise its temperature through 1°F, and to raise the temperature from room temperature, say 62°F, to boiling (212°F), i.e. through 150°F, it will take $5\frac{1}{3} \times 150 = 800$ B.T.U. If we know that the heating power of 1 cubic foot of gas is 400 B.T.U. it is obvious that it will take 2 cubic feet to boil the kettle. In similar fashion it can be discovered how much gas it will take to boil any quantity of water in any size boiler, and if the gas is priced at so much per cubic foot, an approximate estimate of keeping the boiler going can be made.

SPECIFIC HEAT

Mention was made in the foregoing illustration of the 'specific heat' of iron. This needs explanation. It has been said that it takes 1 calorie to raise the temperature of 1 g of *water* through 1°C. It was found upon experiment that no other substance (with the exception of hydrogen under constant pressure) needs quite so much heat to raise its temperature. In other words, substances other than water get hot more quickly than water when subjected to the same heating source. They also cool more quickly when the heating source is removed. The amount of heat that

1 g of a substance needs to raise its temperature 1°C is called its specific heat.

The word specific is a familiar one to nurses. For instance, some diseases are best treated by a drug that has a specific effect on that disease, such as salicylic acid in acute rheumatism, or streptomycin on tuberculosis. Yet again, certain diseases cause certain signs and symptoms that are specific for that disease and occur in no other. Or still further, that antibodies in the blood stream are each specific for a certain antigen and have no effect on any other. So too with the specific heats of substances. Each substance needs a certain amount of heat to raise the temperature of 1 g through 1°C.

Water, by definition, needs 1 calorie for this. Hence its specific heat is 1. If we do some experiments and find that the temperature of 1 g of iron filings is raised by 1°C after supplying it with only 0.125 calories we can say the specific heat of iron is 0.125. The practical application of this is that we can predict the rise in temperature that will result from supplying any weight of any substance with a certain quantity of heat by multiplying the weight by the specific heat and dividing this product into the number of calories supplied.

From a list of some specific heats interesting facts emerge.

Sand	0.19	Water	1.00
Turpentine	0.42	Steel	0.126
Aluminium	0.21	Zinc	0.096
Cast iron	0.125	Copper	0.097
Mercury	0.03	Tin	0.056

The specific heat of sand is 0.19 while that of water is 1. This means that land, particularly land bare of vegetation, will get much hotter than the adjoining water under the action of the sun. It will get five times hotter approximately, or rather, it will get hot five times as quickly. At night it will lose its heat five times faster than the water. Hence the relative coolness of sea breezes during the later part of the day, and the relative warmth of the same breezes in the later part of the night.

Aluminium has a higher specific heat than cast iron, so that if saucepans of these two metals having the same weight are used to boil water, the water in the cast iron one will boil first. In actual practice, however, it is found that aluminium, being so much less dense than cast iron, is more suitable as the saucepans can be made of much thinner metal.

The specific heat of mercury is very low; only 0.03. This means that mercury will absorb heat about thirty-three times faster than water and a simple experiment can be performed to show that this is so.

Take two beakers of the same size and place in one 100 g of water. Place in the other 100 g of mercury. Take the temperatures of both liquids and note them. Place the beakers over bunsen flames of equal size and intensity to ensure as nearly as possible that both liquids are receiving heat at the same rate. Heat for 3 minutes. Take the temperatures of both liquids at the end of this time. Subtract the starting temperatures from the final temperatures to find the rise in both cases and it will be apparent that the mercury has gained approximately thirty-three times as much heat as the water.

From this emerges a very good reason for using mercury instead of water in clinical thermometers. If such a thermometer were filled with water it would take more than half an hour for it to register where the mercury thermometer takes only 1 minute.

Another glance at the list of specific heats reveals that zinc and copper have lower specific heats than steel. This explains why they are often used for making sterilizers. Tin would be even better if it were not for the fact that it melts at a temperature of only 232°C.

LATENT HEAT

Although it takes 1 calorie to raise the temperature of 1 g of water by 1°C, there comes a time when the temperature of the water will rise no further no matter how many more calories are supplied. This point is reached when the water starts to boil and from then on it will stay at a temperature of 100°C while it gradually 'boils away'. In other words, the calories are still being absorbed but they fail to raise the temperature. Instead they provide the energy for the water to change into steam. The number of calories required to change 1 g of a liquid substance into a gas is called the latent heat of that particular substance. To be more accurate, it is called the latent heat of vaporization of that particular substance and this distinguishes it from the amount of heat required to change a solid to a liquid, which is referred to as the latent heat of fusion of the solid. Considerably more calories are required to bring about these changes of state, and an experiment can be done to find out how much is required to change water into steam.

Place 5 g (5 ml) of water in a beaker and take its temperature. Place the beaker over a flame and note carefully how long it takes the water to boil. It will then be at 100°C so there is no need to take the temperature again. Subtract the original temperature from 100 to find the rise in temperature, and this figure multiplied by 5, the weight of the water, will show how many calories have been absorbed altogether. This last figure divided by the time that it took the water to boil will indicate fairly accurately the rate at which the flame is delivering heat. Continue to boil the water with an undiminished flame and note exactly how long it takes to 'boil dry', i.e. how long it takes for the 5 g of water to be evaporated completely into steam. The rate at which heat is being delivered has been discovered so, by multiplying the last time taken by the rate, the total number of calories required to evaporate 5 g of water is determined. Dividing this figure by 5 will tell us how many calories are required to evaporate 1 g and this is the latent heat of vaporization of water.

The completed calculations should look like this:

Weight of water	= 5 g
Initial temperature of the water	= 20°C
Final temperature of the water	= 100°C
∴ increase in temperature	= 80°C
∴ total number of calories delivered	= 80 × 5 calories
	= 400 calories
Time taken to boil the water	= 2 minutes
∴ flame delivers 400 ÷ 2 calories per minute	= 200 calories per minute
∴ time taken to evaporate all the water	= 14 minutes
∴ total heat used to vaporize 5 g of water	= 200 × 14 calories
∴ heat required to vaporize 1 g of water	$= \frac{200 \times 14}{5}$ calories
	= 40 × 14
	= 560 calories

Therefore the latent heat of vaporization of water is 560 by this experiment.

Actually there will be some loss of heat to the beaker and the surrounding air which has not been accounted for, so the real figure is slightly lower at 536. Even so it proves a remarkable point, i.e. that substances need a considerable amount of energy in order to change their state from solid to liquid and from liquid to gas. This extra energy remains locked up in the molecules of the substance until a change takes place back into its original state, whereupon all this energy is released again.

The latent heat of fusion of ice is 80. In other words, ice needs 80 calories per gram to turn into water. It also means that when water turns into ice it *releases* 80 calories per gram. This principle has been used for heating purposes. It is possible to decompress water suddenly so that it turns to ice. The heat liberated from this process is then collected and used for heating air to circulate round buildings.

The very great latent heat of steam explains why a scald with steam is so much worse than one with boiling water. Every gram of steam that condenses to water in contact with the skin liberates 536 calories while that amount of heat would be liberated by 50 grams of hot water while cooling through 10 degrees.

Water evaporating imperceptibly from the skin takes 536 calories per gram just the same as if it were boiling, so nature's mechanism for cooling the blood is a most efficient one.

Exercises

1. If an electric sterilizer containing 6 litres of water takes 20 minutes to boil from an original temperature of 20°C, how long is it safe to leave it before it boils dry? (Take the latent heat of steam to be 540.)

2. How often should a steam kettle containing 2 litres be

refilled if it takes 1 hour for it to boil tap water at a temperature of 15°C?

DIETETIC CALORIES

The normal calorie is far too small a quantity of heat to be of practical value in the study of dietetics, so a more manageable quantity has been devised. This is the 'Large' Calorie and it is the equivalent of 1000 ordinary calories. The dietetic Calorie should always be spelt with a capital 'C' to distinguish it from the small one, but this is often ignored in practice as the large Calorie is the only one used in dietetics and confusion cannot arise provided newcomers to dietetics realize what they are dealing with from the start.

A dietetic Calorie can be defined as the amount of heat needed to raise the temperature of 1 litre of water through 1°C. In the English system it is the amount of heat needed to raise the temperature of 1 lb of water 4°F.

At first glance this seems to have little connection with the metabolism of carbohydrates and fats, but as both these substances are burnt in the body it is convenient to use heat units to measure their usefulness. The process of burning in the body is not greatly different from the burning of carbon compounds outside the body; wax candles, coal, petrol, gas, wood and paraffin are all carbon compounds that utilize oxygen to produce heat energy. Waste products resulting from the combustion include carbon dioxide and water which escape into the air. Inside the body carbohydrates, fats and proteins also utilize oxygen to produce energy with the production of the waste products carbon dioxide and water.

If a controlled experiment takes place, it is found that the oxygen needed to burn a certain amount of carbohydrate outside the body is almost constant, also the amount of carbon dioxide is constant. It is very likely, therefore, that the same definite quantity of oxygen is needed to burn the same amount of carbohydrate inside the body, and the same amount of carbon dioxide is produced. Oxygen intake and carbon dioxide output can be measured readily, and it is indeed found that dietary intake, oxygen intake and carbon dioxide output balance perfectly just as they do outside the body. In the case of carbohydrates catabolism or usage is almost 100%, of fats it is about 95%, and of proteins about 92%, the unburnt portions of the fats and proteins escaping from the body as urea, creatine, uric acid and so on.

The amount of energy being produced inside the body cannot be measured directly, but as long as oxygen intake and carbon dioxide output remain constant factors, it is possible to work out mathematically the energy production. Most of the knowledge that we have regarding dietary requirements has been discovered in this way.

BASAL METABOLIC RATE

Certain body functions such as heart beat, respiration, maintenance of body temperature, circulation of blood and glandular secretion, continue incessantly. These functions represent the absolute minimum activity that is necessary to keep a person alive and the rate at which substances are burnt to maintain these essential functions is termed the basal metabolic rate.

In order to measure this rate, the subject must be at absolute rest and digestion must have ceased. The usual time to take the measurements is first thing in the morning after fasting for at least 12 hours. A spirometer moves up and down as the subject breathes in and out of it, and these movements are recorded on a revolving drum. As the oxygen is used up a curve results, from which the amount of oxygen used is calculated. Carbon dioxide is absorbed into a suitable chemical which is weighed before and after the experiment, the difference in weight representing the amount of carbon dioxide exhaled. The basal metabolic rate is based on the respiratory quotient, which is the figure resulting from dividing the amount of carbon dioxide by the amount of oxygen. If combustion in the body were complete the amount of carbon dioxide produced would be exactly equal to the amount of oxygen taken in and the respiratory quotient would be 1. As proteins and fats are not burned to completion, there is less carbon dioxide exhaled than there is oxygen inhaled so that the respiratory quotient in normal healthy individuals is about 0.85. This represents a Calorie requirement of roughly 1500 for a person of average height and weight, say 175 cm (5ft 9in), and 65 kg (10 stone 4 lb).

In other words the average adult male requires food that will provide him with 1500 Calories merely to remain alive. Anything less in the diet means that he will start using stored glycogen; when that is exhausted, and the maximum amount that can be stored is about 540 grams, the body fats are used, and last of all the tissue proteins. To do any sort of work, even the lightest imaginable, will require food intake over and above that needed to maintain basic metabolism.

Joules

The introduction of S.I. units should have meant that the joule was introduced as the unit of measurement for the energy value of food. However, after much deliberation the Metrication Board decided that the Calorie should be retained. In view of this, it is only necessary to mention the joule in order that you are familiar with the term.

As with calories the joule is too small to be used in

dietetics and so the kilojoule, which is equal to 1000 joules, is used instead:

$$1 \text{ Calorie} = 4.184 \text{ kilojoules}$$
$$\text{and } 1000 \text{ Calories} = 4184 \text{ kilojoules}$$

Table 9 lists a few commonly used foodstuffs with their energy values in both Calories and kilojoules.

Table 9. Calorie and Kilojoule Values per 100 Gram Edible Portion of some Commonly Used Foodstuffs

	Calories	*kilojoules*
Milk (whole)	65	272
Bread (white)	251	1050
Sugar	394	1648
Butter	731	3058
Cheese (Cheddar)	412	1724
Beef	226	946
Apple	46	192
Fish (cod)	76	318

CALCULATION OF INFANT FEEDS

All nurses in training are required to spend a period, if only a brief one, in a paediatric ward. During this time some contact with young babies is inevitable and they do, of course, have to be fed. To most nurses in general training the calculation of infant feeds is one of those mysteries of life which are destined never to be solved.

Many hospitals do, of course, use prepacked feeds, much to the relief of the trainees. However, it is worth remembering that, in the opinion of the public, someone who has trained as a nurse automatically knows everything about babies. It is therefore wise for nurses to familiarize themselves with the rudiments of infant feeding and an attempt has been made here to simplify these as much as possible. It is also worth remembering that most mothers have no special training in calculating feeds and that most babies survive, and so the difficulties cannot be insurmountable.

Basic information required

When calculating infants feeds it is essential to know two basic facts before commencing:

1. The birth weight
2. The age of the baby in weeks.

These are necessary to obtain the *expected weight*, on which the feed will be calculated. A baby should regain his birth weight by the time he is two weeks old, having initially lost anything up to 10% within the first few days of life. This first fortnight is therefore ignored when making the calculation, since a baby of 12 weeks will have actually been gaining for 10 of those. From 2 to 12 weeks a baby should gain about 200 g/week. Therefore, a baby of 12 weeks of age, who weighed 3000 g (3 kg) at birth, would have his expected weight calculated as follows:

Birth weight	= 3000 g
Age	= 12 weeks, from which 2 weeks will be deducted = 10 weeks
Expected gain	= 200 g/week
Thus 200×10	= 2000 g/gained

This is then added to the original weight:

$$2000 + 3000 = 5000$$

$$\therefore \text{ the expected weight} = 5000\text{ g } (5\text{ kg})$$

Calculation of the feed

Having ascertained the expected weight of the baby, one compares it with the actual weight. If he is sick, his weight is probably less than it should be, and one usually attempts to feed him to a level somewhere between his actual and expected weights. Two more factors have now to be considered:

1. Fluid requirements
2. Energy requirements.

Fluid requirement. The normal infant requires

150 to 200 ml/kg body weight/day

Therefore if a baby weighs 4 kg it requires

$$4 \times 150\,\text{ml to } 4 \times 200\,\text{ml/day} = 600\text{–}800\,\text{ml}$$

Energy requirement. The normal infant requires

420 to 540 kJ (100 to 130 Calories)/kg body weight/day

If a baby weighs 4 kg it requires

$$4 \times 420\,\text{kJ to } 4 \times 540\,\text{kJ/day}$$
$$= 1680\text{–}2160\,\text{kJ } (400\text{–}520\text{ Cal})\text{/day}$$

This amount is then divided into evenly spaced feeds of equal amount, e.g. 120 ml four-hourly for five feeds.

Exercises

Using the foregoing information, calculate the following:

1. What are the expected weights of a baby who:
   (*a*) Weighed 2.5 kg at birth and is now 6 weeks old?
   (*b*) Weighed 3 kg at birth and is now 10 weeks old?
   (*c*) Weighed 4 kg at birth and is now 8 weeks old?
2. What are the fluid and energy requirements of the following?

(*a*) A baby of 12 weeks who weighs 5 kg?
(*b*) A baby of 8 weeks who weighs 4 kg?

3. Calculate the feeding requirements for a baby of 10 weeks who weighed 4 kg at birth.

Further calculations

After three months of age the infant gains weight less rapidly. Table 10 gives the approximate amounts for the first two years of life. As the weight gain slows down, so do the fluid and energy requirements per kilogram.

Table 10. Approximate Weight Gain for Infant from 0 to 24 Months

Age (months)	*Weight gain (grams/week)*
0–3	200
3–6	150
6–9	100
9–12	50–75
12–24	2.5 kg during the year

However, the total amount required continues to *increase* as the child grows. Many babies who are very sick need to have their feeds calculated by a dietician, and the information given here applies only to those who do not require special feeds. It should, however, be sufficient to enable a nurse to determine the needs of a normal infant, or give advice to a mother.

14 Pressure and its Effects

The measurement of pressure forms an important aspect of the work of the nurse. It is important, therefore, that she or he is familiar with the underlying concepts. This chapter explains the principles.

Anything resting on a surface exerts a downward force distributed over the resting surface equal to its own weight. A cube of metal weighing 1 kg and with surfaces of 10 sq cm on each side exerts a force of 1 kg over 10 sq cm. This is a *pressure* of (1000 ÷ 10)g on each sq cm, i.e. 100 g per sq cm. Pressure can be defined as force per unit area.

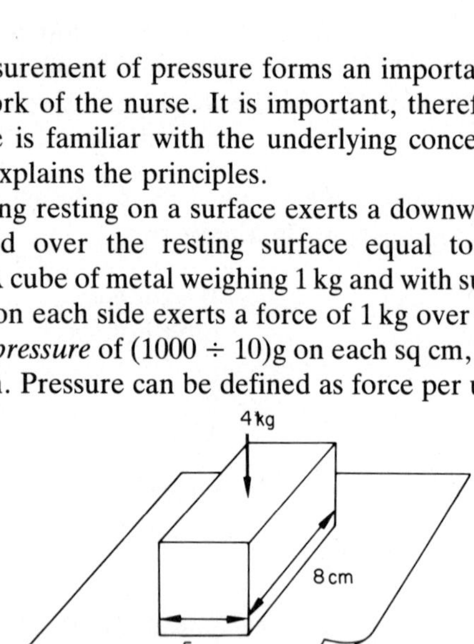

4 kg distributed over an area of
$40\,cm^2 = 100\,g/cm^2$

This example is perfectly straightforward because the solid metal is tangible and solid. It can be weighed easily and the area of its regular sides can be determined easily. When calculating the pressure in liquids the density and depth of the liquid must be known. As liquids are practically incompressible the pressure will increase at a regular rate with the depth. This is expressed technically by saying that the pressure varies directly with the depth.

With gases, however, there are several complicating factors. For one thing, the weight of a gas is not a constant factor. Since gas is compressible a given weight of gas can be made to occupy any desired volume. For instance, a gas cylinder may have an internal volume of 60 litres; into this space it is possible to force 9.36 kg of air so that the air under those circumstances weighs 156 g per litre. If this air is released in an ordinary room it will expand to occupy something like 7200 cubic decimetres so that it weighs approximately 1.3 g per cubic decimetre (litre). The empty cylinder still contains 60 litres of air with a weight of 78 g. If three-quarters of this air is sucked out with a suction pump, the remaining quarter will then expand to fill the available space and its weight will now be 0.325 g per litre. Furthermore the volume and hence the weight of a gas will remain constant only if the temperature remains constant. The volume will increase by $\frac{1}{273}$ for every rise of temperature of 1°C. These difficulties make it impossible to perform accurate and reliable experiments unless complicated equipment is available. Even so, nurses can perform experiments that prove that air has *some* weight, which will prove that it exerts pressure.

Take two compressed air cylinders (oxygen cylinders will do, since the experiment is to prove that gas has weight), one full and unused, the other empty. They should both be the same size. Weigh them and compare the weights. The empty one should weigh much less.

A second experiment can be done this way. Take a large flask fitted with a rubber bung. Place some water in the flask and weigh all together. Remove the bung and boil the water vigorously for a few seconds. The steam from the water will drive out all the air. Remove the flask from the heat and in the same moment replace the bung, thus preventing air re-entering the flask. Let the flask cool thoroughly and weigh again. It will be found that there is a slight loss of weight. As air only weighs 1.3 g per litre under atmospheric pressure and at a temperature of 0°C, the larger the flask used for this experiment the more reliable the results will be.

Having determined that air has weight it must follow that it exerts pressure. Indeed, when one considers that there is an envelope of air around us that is many miles thick, it is not surprising to find that it exerts a pressure of 15 lb to the square inch at sea level (approximately 1 kg per square centimetre). The pressure diminishes as one ascends through the atmosphere, as one would expect. The less air there is above one the less pressure it can exert.

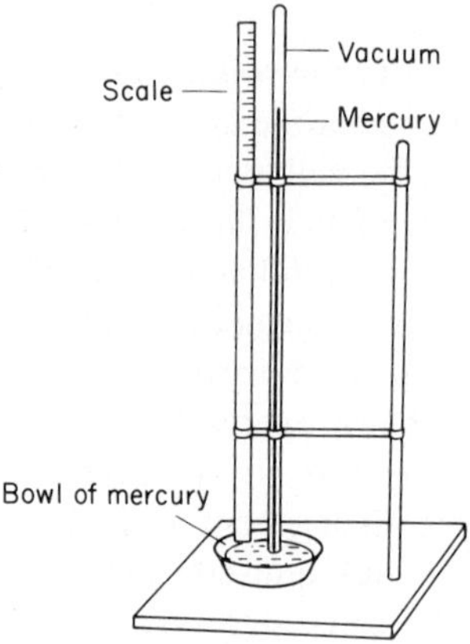

A simple mercury barometer

The barometer is the instrument used for measuring air pressure. It is fairly easy to construct one as it consists of a glass tube about a yard long sealed at one end. This is filled with mercury and inverted into a bowl of mercury. The pressure of the air on the surface of the mercury in the bowl is sufficient to support only about 760 mm of the mercury; at this point the tendency of the air to push mercury up the tube exactly counterbalances the tendency of the mercury to flow out of the tube. As the tube was originally filled and is about 92 cm long, when the tube is inverted some of the mercury will run out leaving a vacuum behind.

If it is desired to find out how long a tube must be to form a water barometer, it can be done mathematically quite easily. The density of mercury is 13.6 grams per cubic centimetre, and atmospheric pressure is 760 mm (76 cm) of mercury. The density of water is 1 gram per cubic centimetre. Therefore it follows that if water is to be used the length of the column would need to be:

$$76 \times 13.6 = 1033.6 \text{ cm}$$

Thus a water barometer tube would have to be at least 10.3 m (33.8 ft) in length.

If the tube of a mercury barometer is fixed in an upright position and a scale fitted alongside, observations can be made over a period to see what variations occur in the height of the mercury. It will be seen that the height is sometimes more than 760 mm and sometimes less, which indicates that the air pressure varies. The explanation for this lies in the fact that air is a mixture of gases and one of these, water vapour, varies in quantity at different times. As water vapour is lighter than dry air when both are at the same temperature and pressure, it follows that a given volume of the air will be lighter the more water vapour it contains. Generally speaking, a fall in barometric pressure indicates a moister atmosphere and one can expect rain. This is not so all over the world, but it is usually the case in England.

Temperature also affects barometric pressure. Air expands as it gets warmer and a given volume will be lighter in consequence. Warm air is capable of containing more water vapour, which will depress the barometer still further.

The effect of pressure on boiling point

Under normal atmospheric pressure water boils at a temperature of 100°C (212°F). Steam issuing from such water is also at a temperature of 100°C (212°F) and is said to be moist or saturated steam. If the pressure is increased, as in a boiler, the boiling point of the water rises. With a pressure of 760 mm × 2 (15 lb above atmospheric pressure = 2 atmospheres) water boils at 121°C (250°F). At 760 mm × 3 (30 lb pressure above atmospheric pressure = 3 atmospheres) the boiling point is 133°C (271.4°F). The steam coming from such water is superheated, or dry steam, and is much used in hospitals and laboratories for sterilization purposes. All ordinary bacteria are killed in seconds by a temperature of 100°C (212°F), but spores may survive after as much as twenty minutes exposure. They are killed by temperatures over 110°C (230°F) and heating in an autoclave is very suitable treatment. A further advantage is that superheated steam will not damage fabrics or cause scorching.

If increasing the pressure raises the boiling point it is reasonable to expect that the reverse is true, as indeed it is. An easy way to reduce the pressure on some water is to boil some in a flask. When it is boiling vigorously the steam will drive out all the air. If the flask is then corked quickly, taking care to remove the source of heat immediately, no air can get in and the water in the flask is no longer subjected to air pressure. If the flask is then held under the cold water tap the contained water will be seen to boil vigorously.

Another way of proving that reduced air pressure lowers the boiling point is to take the temperature of water boiling on the top of a mountain. Attempting to make tea with this boiling water gives quite dramatic proof that it is not as hot as water boiling at the foot of the mountain. This explains perhaps why experienced mountaineers take a pressure cooker as an essential piece of equipment.

Safety valves

The strength of a boiler is the strength of the weakest part of its walls, just as the strength of a chain is the strength of its weakest link. The difficulty with a boiler is to find its weak spots and strengthen them. This is overcome by making the boiler quite a lot stronger than is necessary for the job it has to do and then making a 'weak spot' deliberately. This artificial 'weak spot' is the safety valve. It consists of a metal plug fitting closely into a hole in the top of the boiler. The plug has a definite weight and a definite surface area onto which the pressure of the boiler can exert its force. When the pressure reaches a certain point it overcomes the weight of the plug and pushes it out. Some steam is released, the pressure drops to within the safety margin and the plug falls back into place.

Examples

A boiler is constructed to produce steam at a pressure of 50 lb per sq inch above atmospheric pressure. The safety valve has an internal surface area of $\frac{1}{2}$ sq in. What must its weight be?

$$\begin{aligned} \text{Steam pressure} &= 50\,\text{lb per sq in} \\ \text{Area of safety valve} &= \tfrac{1}{2}\,\text{sq in} \\ \therefore \text{force needed to lift it} &= 50 \times \tfrac{1}{2}\,\text{lb} \\ &= 25\,\text{lb} \end{aligned}$$

$\therefore$ the weight of the safety valve is 25 lb

Another boiler is constructed to produce steam at a

pressure of 3.25 kg per square centimetre above atmospheric pressure. The safety valve has an internal surface area of 2 square centimetres. What must its weight be?

Steam pressure = 3.25 kg/sq cm
Area of safety valve = 2 sq cm
∴ force needed to lift it = 3.25 × 2
= 6.5 kg
∴ weight of the safety valve is 6.5 kg

THE SPHYGMOMANOMETER

The sphygmomanometer is a piece of apparatus for recording blood pressure. It consists of a rubber 'cuff' which can be inflated by means of a rubber bulb-pump connected to the cuff by tubing. A further tube communicates with a mercury pressure gauge or manometer. The cuff is strapped round the patient's arm and sufficient air is pumped into it to compress the blood vessels in the arm. The air is then released, allowing the pressure to fall until the pulse just becomes apparent. The height of the mercury is then noted and this indicates the systolic pressure. This figure is usually expressed in millimetres and sometimes only the figures are written down, thus: 120 or 130.

Often the blood pressure is expressed as a fraction, e.g. 120/80 or 135/86 mmHg (Hg is the chemical symbol for mercury). The top figure is the systolic pressure. The lower figure is called the diastolic pressure and is the pressure existing in the heart and large arteries while the heart is resting between beats. This pressure is not so easy to determine as the systolic pressure and a stethoscope is required. When the diastolic pressure is to be taken, the systolic pressure is taken first, the stethoscope being applied to the bend of the elbow in order to hear when the heart beat recommences. The air pressure is then further reduced until the sound of the heart beat changes to a muffled tone. The manometer will be registering the diastolic pressure when the sound can still just be heard.

THE SYRINGE

One of the commonest instruments depending on air pressure is the syringe. The piston must fit the barrel very closely or the syringe is inefficient. One can explain the action of the syringe by saying that when the piston is withdrawn liquid is 'sucked up' into the barrel. It is more

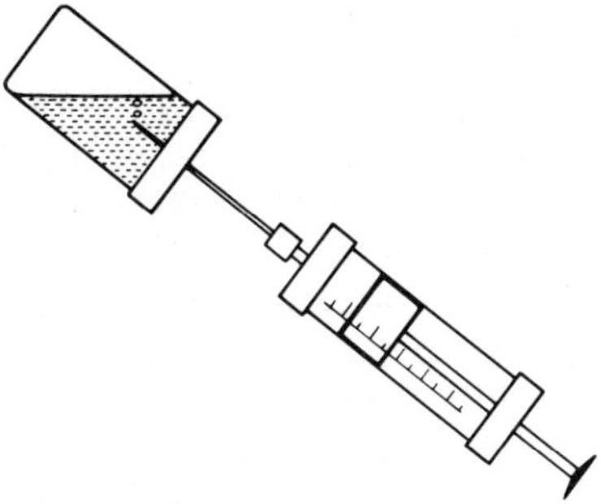

Inject a little air before drawing up

correct to say that when the piston is withdrawn liquid is pushed into the barrel by the pressure of the air on the surface of the liquid outside the syringe. Drawing back the piston reduces pressure inside the syringe while it remains constant outside, and liquids always flow from the high pressure region towards the low.

When a needle is inserted into a vein it is not unusual for the blood to force back the piston of the syringe without the operator having to exert any force. This indicates that the blood in that particular vein is under greater pressure than atmospheric pressure.

Yet again, when extracting liquids from bottles with rubber caps on them it often happens that it becomes difficult to fill the syringe properly. The liquid inside such bottles is not open to the atmosphere, and as one extracts more and more liquid from them the contents remaining are subjected to lower and lower pressure. The point is soon reached where it is impossible to reduce the pressure in the syringe below that in the bottle and the liquid will not flow. This is easily overcome by injecting some air into the bottle beforehand, thus causing a pressure higher than atmospheric. The liquid will then flow into the syringe just as it does from a vein.

THE SIPHON

The easiest way to empty a container of water when it is not supplied with a tap is to siphon the water out. To do this, take a length of wide-bore rubber tubing and fill it with water. Place one end of the tubing below the surface of the water in the container and the other end in a bucket. The water will then flow into the bucket provided the surface of water in the bucket is below that in the container and provided the end in the container stays under water.

Looking at this set-up it will be observed that the water must flow uphill through some part of the tubing, and this needs an explanation.

Air is pressing equally on the surface of the water in the container and on that in the bucket. In both cases there is a tendency for this air pressure to force water up the tube. This tendency is reduced by the water already in the tube tending to flow back into the container on the one hand, and into the bucket on the other. If the tube leading to the bucket is longer than the part leading to the container the water it contains reduces the effectiveness of the air pressure by a greater amount on the bucket side. The effective air pressure is therefore greater on the surface of the water in the container and the water flows into the bucket. If we then raise the bucket from the floor so that it is higher than the container we reverse the position and the water will flow from the bucket back into the container.

The commonest use of the siphon principle in everyday life is the lavatory flush. The pipe leading from the cistern to the pan is empty until the chain is pulled. The act of pulling the chain fills the pipe and, as its end is below the

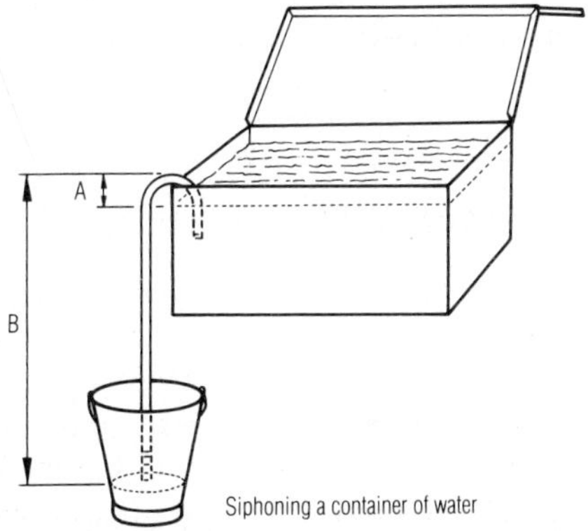

Siphoning a container of water

The tendency of the water to flow into the bucket along 'B' exceeds the tendency of the water to flow back into the container along 'A'

water in the cistern, water flows down to flush the pan. As soon as the water in the cistern falls below the entrance of the pipe, air is sucked in and breaks the siphon. The cistern fills again and is ready for the next occasion when the chain is pulled. The larger the bore of the tube and the greater the height of the cistern above the pan, the more force there is in the water flushing the pan.

RESPIRATION

Respiration is brought about by the alternate increase and decrease of pressure in the thorax above and below atmospheric pressure. When the diaphragm descends and the ribs are raised up by the intercostal muscles, the pressure in the lungs themselves is reduced below atmospheric pressure. Air then flows from the region of higher pressure to that of lower pressure. Expiration takes place when the intrathoracic pressure becomes greater than atmospheric. The difference in pressures required to effect this is surprisingly small. In normal quiet respiration the pressure difference is sufficient to support a column of water about 5 cm high. Compare this with arterial blood pressure which is sufficient to support a column of water 165 cm high.

INTRAPLEURAL PRESSURES

Surrounding the lungs is a double layer of serous membrane called the pleura. The parietal layer is fixed to the chest wall by connective tissue and the visceral layer to the surface of the lung. The two layers are separated by a thin layer of fluid which acts as a lubricant so that the lung can expand and contract without friction. If a needle connected to a 'U' tube manometer is inserted into the space between the layers, the intrapleural space, it is discovered that the pressure in the space is considerably less than atmospheric. It is increased and decreased with inspiration and expiration but remains less than atmospheric at all times. This is sometimes referred to as the 'negative pressure' of the intrapleural space, which, though a contradiction in terms, is quite acceptable as it conveys very well the fact that there is always a suction between the two layers.

There is a good reason why this 'negative pressure' exists. The lung tissue itself is of a balloon-like nature and tends to collapse. The thoracic cage is comparatively rigid. Between the tendency to collapse on one hand, and the tendency to remain rigid on the other, a tension is built up between the two layers of pleura. Because the lung tissue is soft it is prevented from collapsing by this tension or negative pressure. If air enters this space, either by design as in artificial pneumothorax or because of disease as in spontaneous pneumothorax, the tension holding out the lung is destroyed and it collapses.

15 Graphs

Graphs are a means of showing relationships in a pictorial fashion instead of in words or figures. A simple type of graph is the bar or line graph used to show differences in such things as quantity, length, weight, area, volume or practically anything else. Nurses are familiar with this type of graph in the form of intake and output charts. A record is kept of every fluid that passes into the patient's body, whether it is taken orally, rectally or by injection, and entered under *intake*. All urine, vomit, haemorrhage and discharge is measured and recorded under *output*. Each day the amounts are totalled thus:

Mr Jones, 16 October

Intake			*Output*		
Hour		*ml*	*Hour*		*ml*
07.00	tea	140			
08.00	tea	280	07.00	urine	350
08.00	medicine	30	10.00	urine	240
11.00	water	300	11.00	drainage	426
14.00	tea	150	14.00	urine	228
17.00	tea	280	18.00	urine	142
20.00	stout	300	22.00	urine	144
23.00	milk	150			
	Total	1630		Total	1530

The following day a fresh sheet is made out, and so it continues as long as a record is required. Succeeding days may show totals like this:

Date	*Intake (ml)*	*Output (ml)*
October 17	1734	1495
18	2102	1704
19	1591	1000
20	1859	1903
21	2272	1780
22	1875	1648
23	1875	1761
24	2000	2000

In some hospitals this may be regarded as sufficient, but often this information is turned into a pictorial record so that it can be seen at a glance how intake and output compare with each other. This pictorial record is a *bar graph*.

There are three essentials of any type of graph. Without them a graph is unintelligible to everyone except the person who made it. The poorer types of advertisement sometimes attempt to gull the public by exhibiting the sort of thing shown below. It is arrant nonsense, of course, because the graph tells one nothing. It cannot do so. It is meaningless.

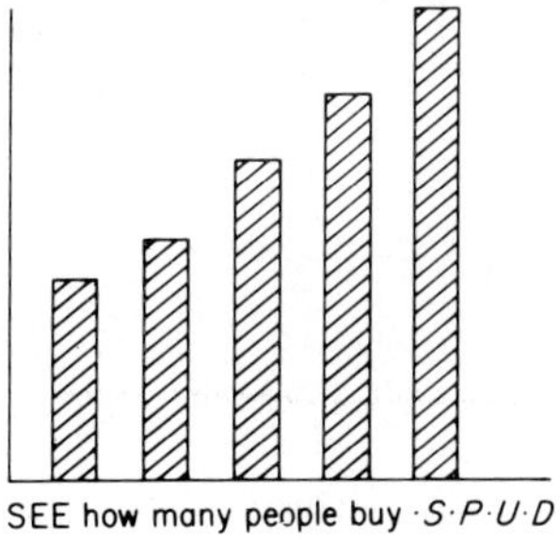
SEE how many people buy ·*S·P·U·D*

Graph 1 shows the three essential features of a bar graph:

1. There must be a vertical scale representing quantity.
2. There must be a horizontal scale representing date.
3. There must be a key whenever two or more things are represented on a graph.

Bar graphs can be drawn on plain paper as in Graph 1, but it saves considerable work and possibility of error if

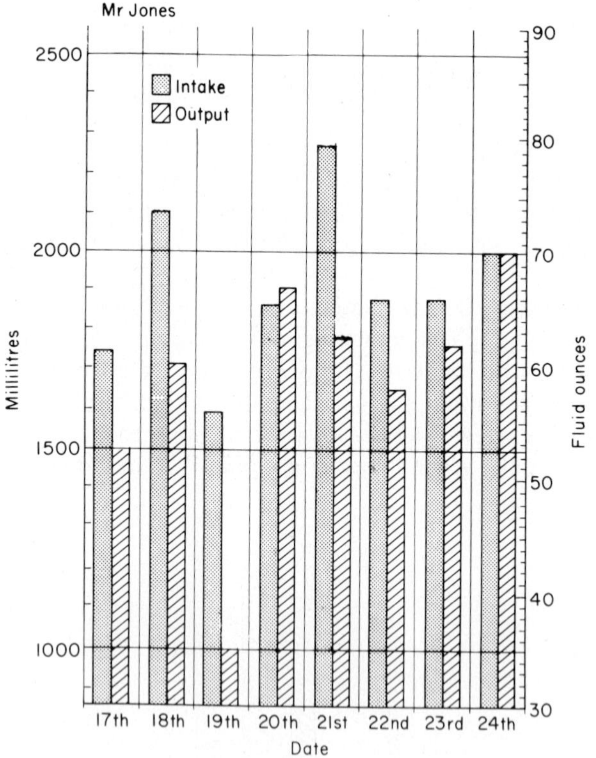

Graph 1

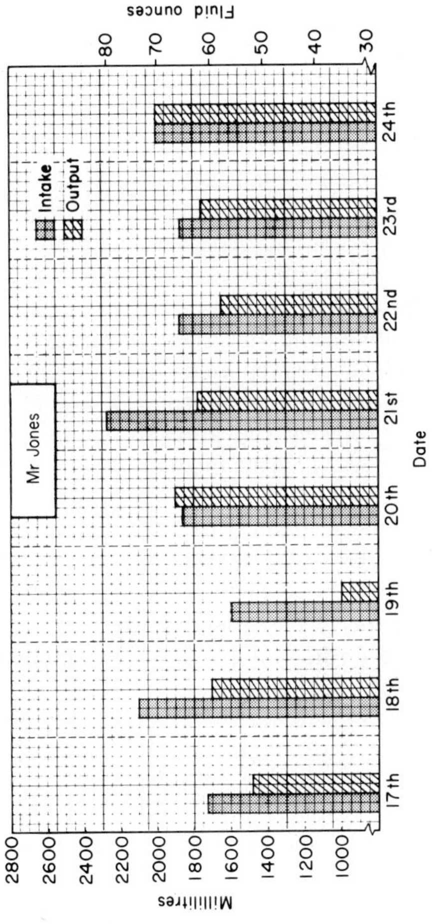
Mr Jones
Intake
Output
Date
17th
18th
19th
20th
21st
22nd
23rd
24th
Millilitres
2800
2600
2400
2200
2000
1800
1600
1400
1200
1000
Fluid ounces
80
70
60
50
40
30

Graph 2

squared paper is used. Plain paper has to be ruled with parallel, vertical and horizontal lines and all this is done ready for use on squared paper. All that remains to be done is to adapt the existing lines to convenient vertical and horizontal *scales*.

A vertical line is drawn towards the left of the paper leaving enough room to be able to write between the line and the edge of the paper. A convenient number of squares are counted off and each small square represents a definite quantity. In Graph 2, the vertical line represents millilitres on the left and ounces on the right. Each small square represents 50 ml.

A horizontal line is similarly drawn leaving sufficient room for writing, and this stands for successive days. Every 10 small squares represents one day. Into this chart is fitted the information gathered each day.

On the 17th (using the previous intake and output record), intake was 1734 ml and output 1495 ml. To represent these quantities on the graph, squares are marked out in proportion to the quantity of fluid taken. Do not forget that the base line of 0 ml is not shown so that only quantities in excess of 800 ml can be indicated on the chart. Alongside the output for the day is similarly indicated. The former column is shaded differently from the latter or blocked out in a different colour to distinguish it. In this example horizontal lines are used for intake and diagonal lines for output. This is repeated each day as the information is gathered and any observer can see all at a glance for the whole of the recorded period.

Another type of graph is the continuous graph, used in nursing mainly in the form of temperature and pulse charts. This type of graph shows the inter-relationship of two different things simultaneously. In the case of the temperature charts it shows the relationship between temperature and time. Each spot on the graph shows two things: (1) the temperature of the patient; and (2) the time the temperature was taken. Successive spots give a clear indication of the 'ups' and 'downs' over a period. This gives immediately a clearer impression to an observer than a simple written list could ever do. The lines drawn connecting the spots make it clearer still.

The same essentials are required for this type of graph as for the bar graph, namely a vertical scale, a horizontal scale, and a key when more than one set of spots are used on the same graph. Squared paper is a useful aid and the temperature charts in use in every hospital are simply a special type of squared paper adapted for that particular form of graph. The vertical and horizontal scales are

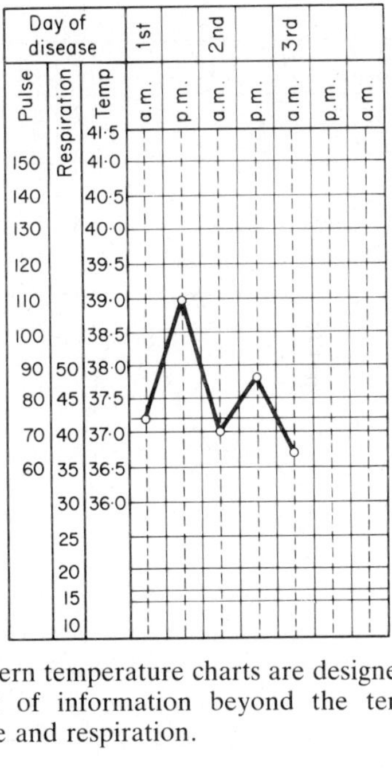

Graph 3. Modern temperature charts are designed to be able to provide a lot of information beyond the temperature; for example, pulse and respiration.

already marked off and space is left for much additional information relevant to any particular patient.

The successive spots marked on a temperature chart are usually joined by straight lines. The lines represent the lapse of time btween successive spots. This interval may be any time at all. It is frequently 12 hours, but can be 6-hourly, 4-hourly or 2-hourly. The commonest in hospitals are morning and evening charts and 4-hourly charts. The temperature in between two successive spots is not known definitely but is inferred to be something in between the temperatures represented by the two spots.

In Graph 3 the first spot represents 37.2°C (99°F) at 06.00 hours on the first day, and the second spot represents 38.8°C (102°F) at 18.00 hours. At 12.00 hours we

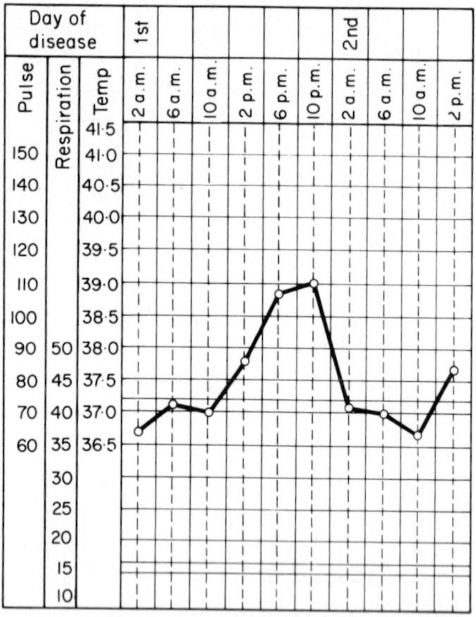

Graph 4. Most temperature charts are so arranged that different time intervals can be used. This sheet is being used as a four-hourly chart.

infer that the temperature was between these two points but we cannot be sure. It could have been something entirely different. If we want to know more accurately we should have to take the temperature at shorter intervals, say 4-hourly. The graph would look something like Graph 4.

This is a good example of the fact that the shorter the interval of time between successive readings, the greater the degree of accuracy obtainable. Sometimes nurses need to have almost a moment to moment account of a patient's condition; for example, during a critical phase such as immediately after an operation when there is a danger of haemorrhage. For this purpose a special type of graph is drawn showing the relationship between pulse rate and time. At 15-minute intervals the pulse is counted and recorded. Graph 5 shows a graph constructed on a 15-minute basis.

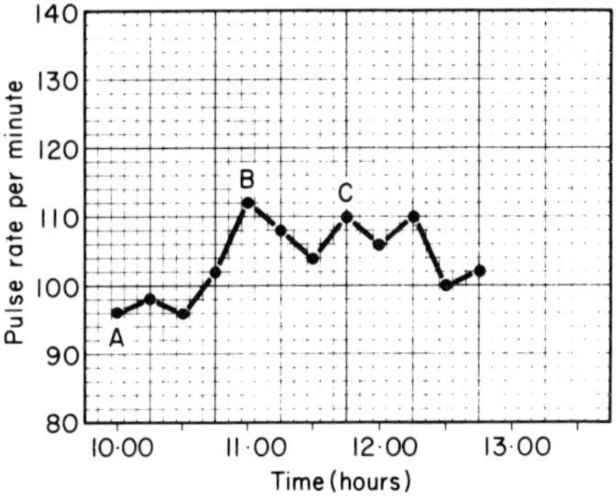

Graph 5

The vertical scale represents pulse rate and extends from 80 per minute at its lowest point to 140 at its highest. This is a range of 60 beats and is spread over 30 small squares. Thus each small square represents 2 beats. The horizontal scale is arranged so that each small square represents 6 minutes so that every two and a half squares mark off a 15-minute period. The spots are placed at the intersections of the relevant vertical and horizontal lines. Spot A represents a pulse rate of 96 because it lies on the horizontal line passing through the scale at 96. It also represents a time of 10.00 hours because it lies on a vertical line passing through 10.00 hours. Similarly spot B represents a pulse rate of 112 at 11.00 hours and spot C 110 at 11.45 hours.

If the interval between recordings was reduced to a negligible period, the spots would be so close together that they would form a continuous line. The individual spots would be unnecessary. Very accurate readings can be taken from continuous line graphs.

An interesting form of continuous line graph is the self-recording pressure graph attached to many autoclaves. These are unusual because they are circular and are rotated by clockwork or electricity. A pen is pressed against the graph paper and a line is traced as the paper rotates. The nib is raised or lowered according to the pressure within the autoclave. Graph 6 shows a simplified diagram of one of these graphs. The radius of the circle takes the place of the vertical scale and the circumference of the circle takes the place of the horizontal scale. In this case the scales represent pressure in pounds per square inch and time in minutes. The line traced in Graph 6 shows that the autoclave was started at A and a partial vacuum was created, until at B the pressure stood at 5 lb per sq in. This was maintained for 5 minutes and at C the pressure started to build up, until at D it reached 30 lb per sq in. Between D and E this pressure was maintained for 20 minutes. From E to F the pressure fell again to 5 lb per sq in, and was maintained at this pressure until G, i.e. for 20 minutes. Thereafter air was admitted until the pressure was atmospheric and the sterilizer was switched off.

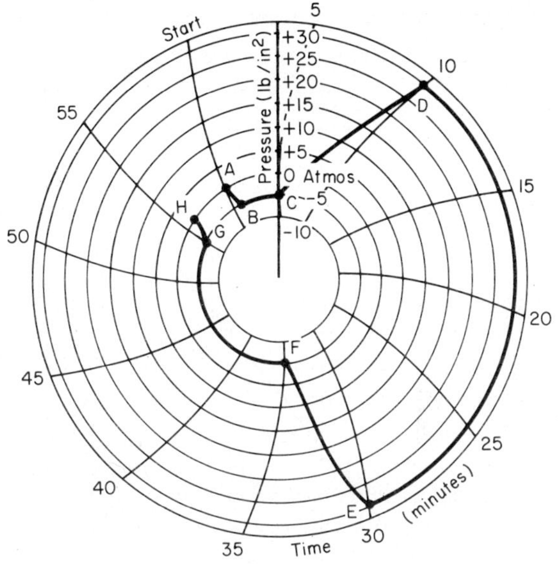

Graph 6. A self-recording pressure graph.

In this way a permanent record can be made every time the autoclave is used and everyone can be sure that the sterilization has been done perfectly.

Now let us construct a graph. A useful one would show the relationship between Celsius and Fahrenheit scales. Instead of having to work out a piece of arithmetic each time we need to convert from one scale to another, all we will need to do is to look up the temperature on one of the scales and see what point corresponds to this on the other scale.

In Graph 7 the horizontal line represents the Celsius scale and shows temperatures between 0° and 110°, a range of 110° over 55 small squares so that each small square represents 2 degrees. The vertical line represents the Fahrenheit scale and shows temperatures between 30°

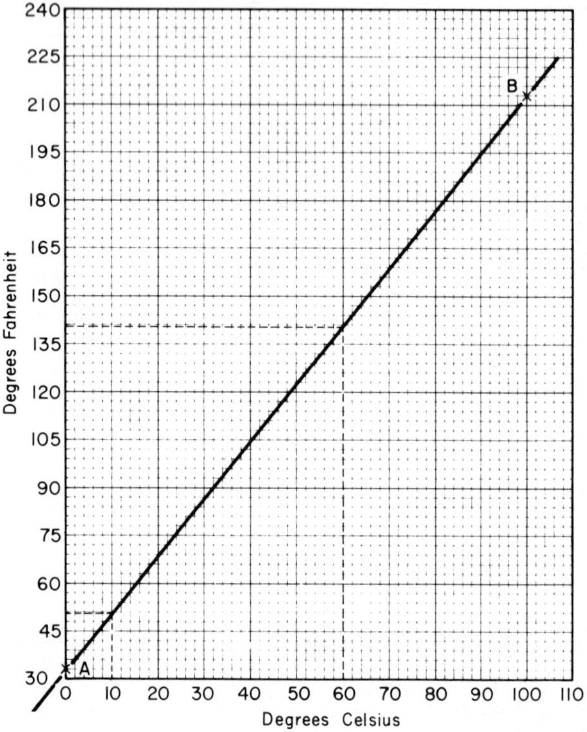

Graph 7. Conversion from Celsius to Fahrenheit and *vice versa*.

and 240°, which is 210 degrees covering 70 small squares so that each small square represents 3 Fahrenheit degrees.

We know that 0°C equals 32°F because that is the freezing point of water, so we can put a cross to show this at A. We also know that the temperature of boiling water is 100° on the Celsius scale and 212° on the Fahrenheit. If we place a cross at B it stands for both these temperatures simultaneously. A line joining A and B completes the graph. The following examples are worked in this fashion.

Look up the temperature 50°F along the vertical scale.

A line is extended horizontally from this point to meet the graph line. From the point where it cuts the graph line a line is extended to the horizontal scale and the temperature read where it cuts the horizontal scale. This is the temperature in degrees Celsius, i.e. 10°C. Actual extension lines have been drawn in this case but it is sufficient to place a ruler on the graph and imagine the lines.

The second example shows how to convert Celsius degrees to Fahrenheit. 60°C is located on the horizontal scale. A line is projected from this point to cut the graph. From the point where it cuts the graph a second line is projected horizontally until it meets the vertical scale. At this point the temperature is read off. It is 140°F.

Exercises

1. With the aid of Graph 7 convert the following Celsius degrees to the Fahrenheit scale: 60, 5, 20, 35, 66, 68, 75, 92.

2. Convert the following Fahrenheit degrees to the Celsius scale: 50, 45, 72, 96, 108, 127, 138, 200, 98.4.

3. Check each one of these by arithmetic.

Example

Construct a graph from the following data showing the relationship between age and weight in an average child during the first 4 months of life.

The vertical line represents weight and extends from 3 kg which is a little below requirements to 6 kg which is a little above. This range of 3 kg extends over 60 small squares so that each square represents 0.05 of a kilogram. The horizontal line stands for age. 16 weeks are represented by 40 small squares so that one week is represented by $2\frac{1}{2}$ small squares.

The information is charted carefully until a series of

Age in weeks	*Weight in kg*
0	3.29
1	3.06
2	3.27
3	3.52
4	3.63
5	3.81
6	3.97
7	4.13
8	4.31
9	4.54
10	4.74
11	4.94
12	5.08
13	5.26
14	5.53
15	5.81
16	5.99

crosses result. These are joined by straight lines. Point A occurs where '0' on the age line intersects 3.29 kg on the weight line. Point B occurs where '1' on the age line intersects 3.06 kg on the weight line, and so on.

From Graph 8 find the following information:

1. Did the baby make up her birth weight in 2 weeks?
2. What was the weight at $8\frac{1}{2}$ weeks?
3. How old was the baby when she weighed 3.72 kg?
4. Did she double her birth weight under the observation period?
5. Did the baby lose weight at any time?

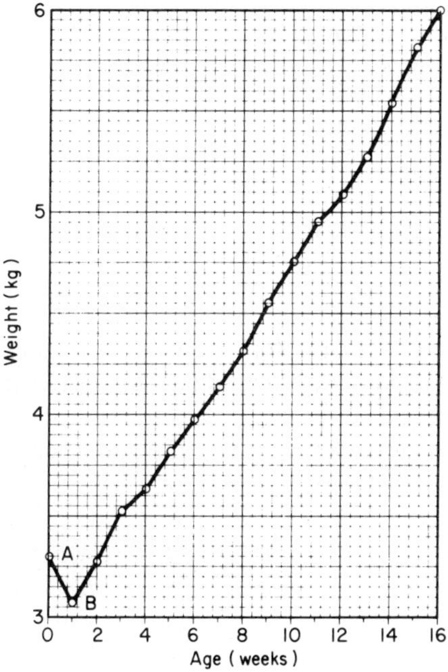

Graph 8. Change in weight of an average baby from 0 to 16 weeks.

Exercises

1. Make a temperature chart using squared paper to include the following:

1st day		*2nd day*		*3rd day*		*4th day*		*5th day*		*6th day*		*7th day*	
a.m. °C	p.m. °C	a.m. °C	p.m. °C	a.m. °C	p.m. °C	a.m. °C	p.m. °C	a.m. °C	p.m. °C	a.m. °C	p.m. °C	a.m. °C	p.m. °C
36.4	37.2	36.6	37.4	36.1	37.8	37.2	38.5	37.6	37.6	37.0	37.5	36.1	37.2

2. Make a temperature chart using squared paper to show the following information. Figures given are degrees Fahrenheit.

Time	*Day 1*	*Day 2*	*Day 3*
02.00	98.4	102.2	101.0
06.00	98.0	99.4	99.2
10.00	98.2	99.0	99.0
14.00	99.0	100.2	99.4
18.00	101.6	102.4	100.0
22.00	102.0	102.0	100.2

3. Construct a blank for recording the pulse rate at 15-minute intervals, in readiness for a patient returning from theatre, to extend over 12 hours.
4. Make a bar graph to show the following intake and output over 1 week:

Day	*Intake (ml)*	*Output (ml)*
1	1320	1180
2	1380	1180
3	1200	1240
4	1560	1360
5	1440	1360
6	1140	1240
7	1800	1550

5. Graph 9 is a graph showing pulse and temperature together from the same patient.
   (*a*) What was the temperature and pulse rate at 'A'?
   (*b*) What was the temperature and pulse rate at 'B'?
   (*c*) When the temperature was 100°F what was the pulse rate?
   (*d*) When the pulse rate was 100 beats per minute what was the temperature?

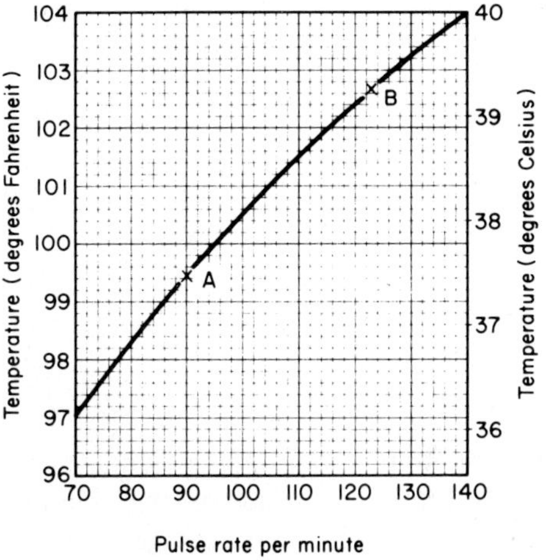

Graph 9

6. Construct a bar graph showing the following rainfall month by month:

January	3.7	February	0.8	March	1.8
April	2	May	3.4	June	1.2
Jule	1	August	nil	September	0.4
October	3.6	November	2	December	2.2

(*a*) What was the total rainfall?
(*b*) What was the average rainfall?
(*c*) Which was the wettest month?
(*d*) Which was the driest month?

7. Draw a graph showing the relationship of weight and age in an average male of height 175 cm using the following information:

Age	*Weight (kg)*	*Age*	*Weight (kg)*
16	61.7	32	69.9
18	63.5	34	70.3
20	65.3	36	70.7
22	66.2	38	71.2
24	67.1	40	71.7
26	68.0	42	72.1
28	68.5	44	72.6
30	68.9	46	73.0

8. On the same graph as the previous question show the following information which is the relationship between age and weight in an average woman of height 160 cm.

Age	*Weight (kg)*	*Age*	*Weight (kg)*
16	50.3	32	55.8
18	51.7	34	56.7
20	52.6	36	57.1
22	53.0	38	57.6
24	54.0	40	58.5
26	54.4	42	59.0
28	54.8	44	59.9
30	55.3	46	60.3

16 Statistics

Although a full treatment of the science of statistics is beyond the scope of this book, a brief study of some of the methods used by statisticians is worth while. We often ask or are asked questions with statistical implications. For example: 'Why do pupils in one school always get better results in examinations than pupils in a similar school down the road?' Is the incidence of a certain disease increasing? If so, to what extent? Do many old people fail to get a balanced diet because protein foods are so expensive? These and many other matters are frequent topics of discussion. Many opinions are expressed, sometimes cogently, but little information of real value can emerge from such discussion unless reliable facts are available to the participants.

Statistics is partly the science of collecting and summarizing facts which can be expressed in numerical form; it is concerned also with the measurement and comparison of facts to try to discover the existence of significant relationships, to reveal trends and so to assist those charged with responsibility for making estimates or forecasts.

THE NORMAL CURVE

If data on a research subject were obtained from the whole of the population of a country, for example information on physical attributes, it would be possible to tabulate the information and arrive at average values for each attribute. Let us consider height. From the mass of information received we would find that most people would be of average height or very near it; the number of people deviating from the average would become progressively smaller as we look towards the extremes of very short and very tall. This is shown in the diagram below.

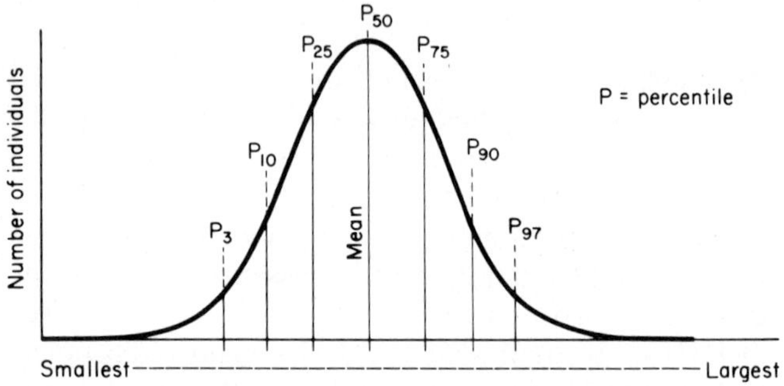

Key : 3rd to 97th percentile – 94% of all individuals
10th to 90th percentile – 80% of all individuals
25th to 75th percentile – 50% of all individuals

Normal distribution of body length

The curve shows the normal distribution of the body length of a large number of people. It will be seen that the numbers at each extreme are similar and that the great majority of people are in the middle ranges. This is an example of *the normal curve.*

Statisticians work on the assumption that given a sufficiently large sample the probability is that the distribution of values will follow the distribution shown on a normal curve. In practice it is rarely possible to obtain information from such large numbers of people and it is necessary to take samples, that is, information from a comparatively small proportion of the populace. If the results of statistical work are to be reliable the opinion of a good cross-section of the population must be obtained.

Special techniques are used to avoid, or to try to avoid, any bias which would unfairly influence and therefore invalidate the results of research. Imagine the results of an enquiry aimed at making a forecast of the results of a general election if people having allegiance to only one of the political parties were questioned! Could the findings be free of prejudice? Alternatively, imagine trying to obtain a reliable sample by taking every fifth name in the telephone directory. This would seem, on the surface, to be a good way of obtaining a random sample, but what about the large number of people who cannot afford or who do not want a telephone? A moment's reflection will reveal that such a sample would not be representative. Everyone should always examine statistical information very carefully to ascertain the source of information and to see what the compiler is attempting to portray. It should be noted that the word 'population' is often used in statistics to describe a group of people who are the subject of a particular piece of research.

SYMBOLS

A brief description of some of the symbols commonly used in statistics is given below, although few symbols are used in this chapter. They are merely a shorthand method of writing expressions which are very long and cumbersome if written in full.

Σ = the sum (addition) of a series of figures. It is the Greek character—large sigma—the equivalent of our S
x = the individual items in a series
$\bar{x}$ = the arithmetic mean
N or n = total frequencies
f = frequency

a = assumed mean
d = deviations from the assumed mean
Q = Quartile. The quarters are usually written as Q_1 for the lower quartile ($\frac{1}{4}$) and Q_3 for the upper quartile ($\frac{3}{4}$).

SOURCES OF INFORMATION

An adequate amount of information must be gathered before any figures can be scientifically treated and meaningful relationships deduced. If the sets of numbers are too small it would be most unwise to draw an inference from the results. At times the information has to be obtained direct from people using techniques such as postal questionnaires or personal interviews; this information is called primary data. Information already available in reports, articles or other published work is called secondary data.

TABULATION

Once the required data have been obtained the groups of facts to be treated are extracted and placed in some order so that they become easier to grasp and manipulate; this process is called tabulation. For example, consider the table below showing the length of time spent in hospital by a hypothetical group of patients.

Number of days spent in hospital by a group of 55 patients

12	20	11	9	8	15	8	5	14	11	21
27	2	17	7	15	10	19	13	17	3	23
3	14	7	11	17	4	13	18	2	15	21
16	17	13	19	14	12	18	6	12	18	22
15	14	6	13	9	16	12	11	25	16	23

It is difficult to see any significance in these figures until they have been rearranged and the frequency of particular numbers can be clearly seen. To achieve this object the numbers have been rearranged in the table below.

Days	*Frequency*	*Days*	*Frequency*	*Days*	*Frequency*
1	0	11	4	21	2
2	2	12	4	22	1
3	2	13	4	23	2
4	1	14	4	24	0
5	1	15	4	25	1
6	2	16	3	26	0
7	2	17	4	27	1
8	2	18	3	28	0
9	2	19	2	29	0
10	1	20	1	30	0

Now a definite pattern is beginning to emerge. If we go a step further and arrange the numbers in groups with a suitable class interval, an impression can be obtained at a glance.

Number of days in hospital	*Number of patients*
1 to 4 days	5
5 to 8 days	7
9 to 12 days	11
13 to 16 days	15
17 to 20 days	10
21 to 24 days	5
25 to 28 days	2
Total	55

It is apparent that the class interval selected is four days and that the majority of the hypothetical patients stayed in hospital for 13 to 16 days. The column is reproduced again below with a third column added showing the cumulative frequency. This column is sometimes used to help show at a glance the proportion or percentage above or below a given value.

Number of days in hospital	*Number of patients*	*Cumulative frequency*
1 to 4 days	5	5
5 to 8 days	7	12
9 to 12 days	11	23
13 to 16 days	15	38
17 to 20 days	10	48
21 to 24 days	5	53
25 to 28 days	2	55
Total	55	

The numbers in the third column are obtained by means of simple addition of the numbers in the second column, the product each time being placed under cumulative frequency. Thus 5 + 7 = 12, 12 + 11 = 23, and so on. The table shows, for example, that 23 people stayed in hospital for less than 13 days, whereas only 17 stayed in hospital for more than 16 days. When a table contains a long list of figures a cumulative frequency column can be a very useful asset.

DIAGRAMS

Diagrams of various types are often used in statistics as a simple but effective means of conveying an instant impression of information gleaned from groups of figures. A histogram is a popular form of diagram, in which the areas within blocks represent the frequencies of particular values. If we use our group of 55 patients just once more we can make a histogram showing the length of stay in hospital, as shown below.

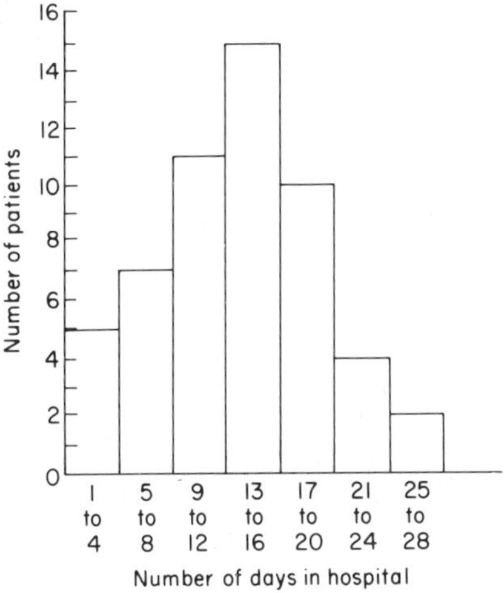

Histogram showing the length of stay in hospital of a group of 55 patients.

Histograms can be used without the ordinate (the vertical line) and abscissa (the horizontal line) being drawn if values are written into the blocks.

PIE CHARTS

A pie chart may be used to represent variable quantities, although the number of quantities shown should not be too many if the diagram is to be effective. The chart is based on a circle so all the quantities together will be represented by the whole 360° of the circle. Each quantity is calculated as a proportion of the whole (in terms of a number of degrees) and is shown as a segment of the pie chart. Let us take as an example a nurse who expects to travel about 10 000 miles a year and who is seeking advice on the cost of running a new car. The dealer may give information a follows:

Estimated annual cost of motoring (10 000 miles)

	£
Petrol and oil	400
Tyres and brake maintenance	40
Servicing charges	200
Depreciation	620
Insurance	100
Road tax	80
	1440

If the dealer has many similar enquiries he may construct a pie chart that will give the required information quickly and is easily comprehended. A small calculation is needed

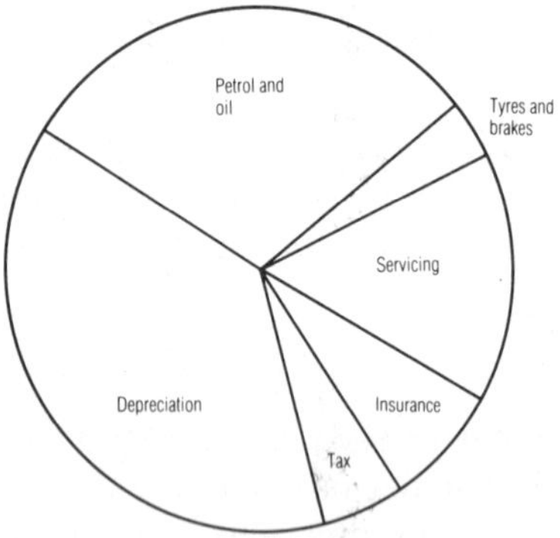

Pie chart showing the cost of motoring 10 000 miles in one year.

to decide the size of each segment. £400 would be given a segment of:

$$400 \times \frac{360}{1440} = 100°$$

Therefore £400 would be represented by 100° of the circle. A similar calculation is carried out for each of the other values. The pie chart would be constructed as shown opposite.

BAR DIAGRAMS

Bar diagrams are also useful for illustrating information in an effective manner. The bars may be drawn vertically or horizontally; the choice depends on whichever is thought to have the greatest visual impact (see page 164).

GRAPHS

Many business people use graphs to show the rate of increase or decrease of their sales as they are particularly suited to this purpose. In a similar way some hospital authorities use them to plot the rates of admission and discharge of their patients. Variables which are measured at regular intervals are known as time series. An example is given in Table 11 which shows the total number of people attending and the total number passing the State final examinations between February 1978 and October 1981.

It is not easy to see a definite pattern by simply looking at the figures, but if they are shown on a graph they have meaning (Graph 10).

Obviously there is little hope of plotting numbers to the nearest unit on a graph of this size, so the figures have become approximate to the nearest fifty. However, the

Table 11. Student nurses who attended and passed the State Final Examination from February 1978 to October 1981

	Attended	*Passed*
February 1978	7617	5392
June 1978	5765	3844
October 1978	8156	5439
February 1979	7874	5164
June 1979	5724	3847
October 1979	7709	5226
February 1980	7504	4698
June 1980	5491	3772
October 1980	7719	5567
February 1981	7488	5298
June 1981	5383	3697
October 1981	7939	5433

Source: The General Nursing Council

graph serves its purpose of giving an immediate overall view of the increase and decrease of attendance and pass rates over the 4-year period.

AVERAGES

We have seen how tabulation and diagrammatic representation can aid the understanding of available data. Now we shall see how the determination of averages provides further description of a collection of figures and helps to bring out the salient points.

The arithmetic mean, median and mode are the averages most commonly used in statistics; the harmonic and geometric averages belong to a more advanced study of the subject.

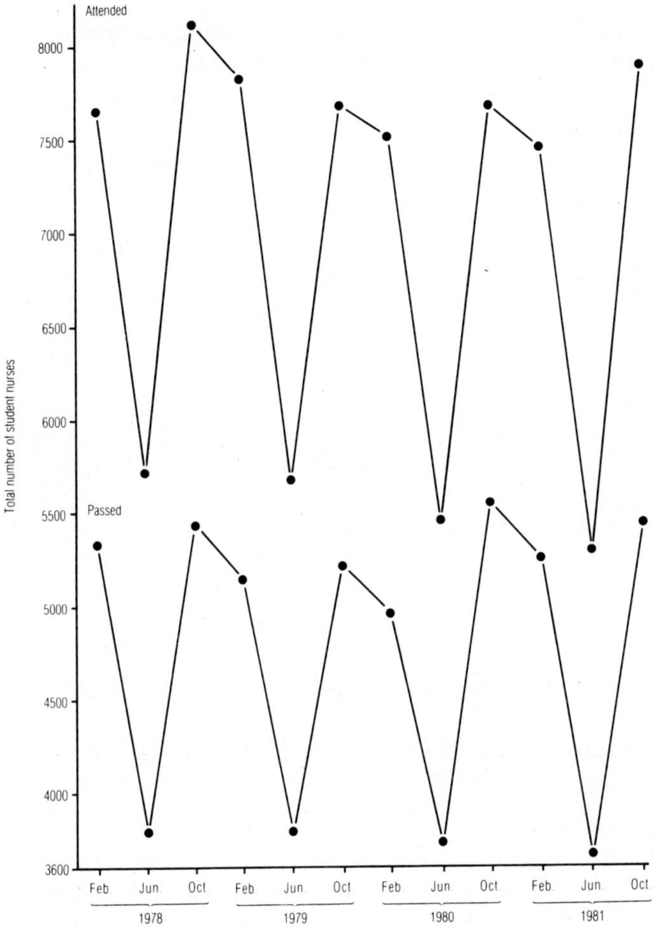

Graph 10. The total number of Student nurses who attended and passed the State Final Examination 1978–81. *Source:* The General Nursing Council.

Arithmetic mean

An arithmetic mean is obtained by dividing the sum of a series of values by the number of values. This is the measure to which most people refer when they speak of 'average'.

Example 1

Eight people pay weekly rent of £20.50, £22.40, £25.00, £27.20, £30.00, £24.50, £23.00 and £26.20, respectively. What is the mean amount of rent?

The total paid is:

£
20.50
22.40
25.00
27.20
30.00
24.50
23.00
26.20
198.80

$$\therefore \text{ the arithmetic mean will be } \frac{198.80}{8} = £24.85$$

When a number of values recur a frequency table can be constructed before the arithmetic mean is calculated.

Example 2

During a 31-day period a casualty department treats numbers of patients for minor injuries, as shown in the following chart. What is the arithmetic mean?

The numbers are first arranged according to frequency, and the number of days is then multiplied by the respective frequency to obtain the total number of patients treated. Note the symbols (x), (f) and ($x \times f$); these signify the number of items (x) and the frequency (f).

Day	*No.*	*Day*	*No.*	*Day*	*No.*
1	55	11	23	21	58
2	25	12	44	22	18
3	18	13	18	23	44
4	21	14	55	24	20
5	32	15	47	25	21
6	23	16	25	26	23
7	70	17	18	27	18
8	18	18	20	28	55
9	25	19	23	29	47
10	21	20	32	30	20
				31	23

Therefore the average number of injuries treated each day over a 31-day period was 31.

Number of incidents per day (x)	*Frequency (numbers of days) (f)*	*Total number of incidents (x × f)*
18	6	108
20	3	60
21	3	63
23	5	115
25	3	75
32	2	64
44	2	88
47	2	94
55	3	165
59	1	59
70	1	70
	31	961

$$\text{Arithmetic mean } \frac{961}{31} = 31$$

A short method of finding the arithmetic mean can be used when the number of values is large. The first step is to arrange the values in ascending order and then the frequency of each number is written in a parallel column. From a study of the numbers so displayed an estimate of the probable arithmetic mean is made. If the values in the first column involve a range, a third column is written giving the mid-point of each range. Thus for a range of 1 to 9 years the mid-point will be 5 years. If decimal values would be inappropriate, ranges such as 1 to 10 should be avoided. Having progressed so far, another column is added for deviations from the assumed mean; for this purpose a class interval can be used if all the values are in proportion to each other.

Example 3

Determine the average age of a group of 100 nurses.

Age range (years)	*Number of nurses (f)*	*Mid-point (x)*	*Deviation (d)*	*Deviation class interval* $\left(\frac{d}{c}\right)$	*Frequency* $\times \frac{d}{c}$ $\left(f \times \frac{d}{c}\right)$
21 to 25	24	23	−15	−3	−72
26 to 30	10	28	−10	−2	−20
31 to 35	12	33	−5	−1	−12
36 to 40*	14	38	0	0	0
41 to 45	14	43	+5	+1	−14
46 to 50	8	48	+10	+2	+16
51 to 55	11	53	+15	+3	+33
56 to 60	7	58	+20	+4	+28
	100				+91
					−104
					−13

*The assumed mean = 38 years

Note:

1. The first two columns are self-evident. The mid-point values of each range in the first column have been placed in the third column (x).
2. Columns 3(x), 4(d) and 5(d/c) are really all related. To obtain the deviation column the assumed mean has been deducted from each mid-point value. As there is a class interval of 5 the numbers can be reduced still further by dividing each deviation by 5.
3. The last column is obtained by multiplying the number of nurses in each range by d/c, e.g. $24 \times -3 = -72$. This is obviously easier and quicker than multiplying 24 $\times$ 23. The whole point of obtaining columns d and d/c is to reduce the amount of tedious counting.
4. Now that column $f(d/c)$ has been completed, add and subtract the numbers as indicated by the signs. Thus: $+91 - 104 = -13$.
5. The true arithmetic mean is found by means of the following formula:

$$\bar{x} = a + \left(\frac{c \times \sum f \frac{d}{c}}{n} \right)$$

Key: $\bar{x}$ = arithmetic mean; a = assumed mean; c = class interval;

$\sum$ = the sum of; f = frequency; d = deviation; n = total frequency;

$\sum f \frac{d}{c}$ = the sum of frequency multiplied by (deviation divided by class interval)

On substituting numbers for the symbols we have:

$$\text{true arithmetic mean} = 38 + \left(\frac{5 \times -13}{100}\right)\text{years}$$

$$= 38 + \left(\frac{-65}{100}\right)$$

$$= 38 + (-0.65)$$

$$= 38 - 0.65$$

$$\therefore \text{the mean} = 37.35 \text{ years}$$

The median

Sometimes the arithmetic mean can be influenced by a very high or a very low figure in a series. Consider, for example, fifteen men whose weekly earnings amount to the following sums: £67, £70, £75, £75, £75, £75, £76, £76, £78, £78, £80, £80, £82, £85 and £90. The arithmetic mean would be

$$\frac{1162}{15} = £77.47$$

This seems to be a reasonable average, but if, in addition, another four men whose earnings are £150, £192, £200 and £250 a week are considered, the arithmetic mean would be

$$\frac{1954}{19} = £102.84$$

The average has obviously been distorted by the high earnings of only four men.

To help correct the distorting effect of extreme values on an arithmetic mean, the median value can be selected. The median (or middle) value is easily obtained when there is an odd number of values in a series; in such cases there will be an equal number of values above and below the median value. It is obtained by the formula:

$$\frac{N + 1}{2}$$

where N equals the number of values. Thus in the above example the median value will be:

$$\frac{19 + 1}{2} = \frac{20}{2}$$
$$= 10$$

The tenth value in the series is £78. If the list is checked we will find nine values above and nine values below the median:

$$\underbrace{67 \quad 70 \quad 75 \quad 75 \quad 75 \quad 75 \quad 76 \quad 76 \quad 78}_{\text{1 to 9}} \qquad \underset{\text{10th}}{\overset{78}{\uparrow}}$$

$$\underbrace{80 \quad 80 \quad 82 \quad 85 \quad 90 \quad 150 \quad 192 \quad 200 \quad 250}_{\text{11–19}}$$

Clearly the median value of £78 is a more accurate portrayal of average earnings than the arithmetic mean of £108.

When there is an even number of values the median is obtained by adding the two middle values and dividing by two. To obtain the median of the numbers 100, 160, 180 and 190, the formula

$$\frac{N + 1}{2}$$

is again used:

$$\frac{4 + 1}{2} = 2.5$$

The half indicates that the median is between the second and third value, therefore the median is

$$\frac{160 + 180}{2} = 170$$

If data have been arranged in groups as shown in the table of nurses' ages, the formula for the median is

$$\frac{N}{2} = \frac{\text{Number of values}}{2}$$

Thus the median age would be $\frac{100}{2} = 50$. That is the age of the fiftieth nurse (which appears to have been 36).

To return to the series of weekly earnings, by taking the division process further we can arrive at the middle values in the ranges above and below the median; these are called quartiles. The first quartile is obtained by the formula

$$\frac{N + 1}{4} = \frac{19 + 1}{4}$$

$$= 5$$

Therefore the first quartile (Q_1) is the fifth value in the series, which is £75. The third quartile is obtained by the formula

$$\frac{3(N + 1)}{4} = \frac{3(19 + 1)}{4}$$

$$= \frac{60}{4}$$

$$= 15$$

Therefore the upper quartile is the fifteenth value, which is £90. Whenever the division yields odd quarters the quartile value is taken to be the nearest whole value. The formulae

$$\frac{N}{4} \quad \text{and} \quad \frac{3N}{4}$$

are used when grouped data are being considered. Statisticians sometimes take these calculations even further to obtain deciles (tenths) and percentiles (hundredths) using the formulae

$$\frac{N}{10} \quad \text{and} \quad \frac{N}{100}\text{, etc.}$$

The mode

The mode is the most frequently occurring value in a series. This kind of average is particularly useful to clothing and shoe merchants; their average sizes are those for which the demand (and sales) are highest. One more reference to the series of weekly earnings will show that the mode for that series is £75.

Summary

From a study of the averages described and the range of values it is possible for the spread of a series to be observed and measured. Knowledge of the spread, sometimes called scatter or dispersion, examined by the use of techniques which determine, for example, the mean deviation and standard deviation, is helpful to enable statisticians to interpret the available data.

INDEX NUMBERS

Before leaving the subject of statistics it is helpful to take a brief look at index numbers. These are the basis of commonly quoted (or misquoted) estimates such as the index of retail prices, popularly known as the cost of living index, or for medical purposes the standardized mortality ratio.

First a base year is selected; the value given to each item in that year will be equated to an index figure of 100. The value of these items in other years is compared with the value in the base year as in the following example.

Example

Standard mortality ratios in males. 1968 = base year

Cause	*1961*	*1968*	*1970*
Tuberculosis	174	100	73
Leukaemia	90	100	96
Poliomyelitis	538	100	110

It can be seen that the figures for 1961 and 1970 indicate the relative increase or decrease in mortality as compared with the base year. A new base year is chosen when the numbers get too high and become unwieldy.

This account of statistics has, of necessity, been very brief. However a number of interesting books are available, such as *Use and Abuse of Statistics* by W.J. Reichmann and *Britain in Figures: A Handbook of Social Statistics* by Alan F. Sillitoe (Pelican Original). A further study of this subject is worth undertaking.

Exercises

1. Determine the number of staff in your hospital or unit, as follows:
   (*a*) Nursing officers and above
   (*b*) Ward sisters and charge nurses
   (*c*) Staff nurses and enrolled nurses

(*d*) Student and pupil nurses
(*e*) Unqualified staff, e.g. ward orderlies or nursing assistants.
Calculate each of these groups as a percentage of the whole and use the percentages to construct a pie chart. What conclusions can you draw from the chart?

2. Ascertain the age of all the patients in your ward. What is the arithmetic mean age? How does the mean compare with the median age and the mode?
3. Record the length of stay of patients in your ward or unit. Prepare a frequency table, using a suitable class interval and from this draw a histogram. What conclusions can you draw?
4. Find out the average daily cost of keeping patients in your hospital and the average length of stay from the records office. Using these averages as a guide estimate the average cost of the care and treatment given to patients admitted and discharged whilst you were working in one of the wards. Compare the hospital and the ward averages.
5. From a published list of examination results in your school of nursing obtain the marks awarded to all the candidates. Prepare a cumulative frequency table from the figures obtained and plot these onto a graph. From the graph calculate, to the nearest whole mark, the median and quartile scores.

17 Computers and the Binary Number System

Computers are being used to an increasing extent in the hospital service and, no doubt, this trend will continue. Many hospitals already have their financial work and other data processed by computers. Some computers are being used as a valuable aid to nursing supervision. In intensive care units, for example, small supervisory systems may be installed to 'watch' body functions such as blood pressure, temperature, respiration, cardiac rhythm (ECG) and brain activity. All these body measurements are fed into a device called a multiplexer and then into a type of computer that has a memory bank of about 12 000 words and which can process $\frac{3}{4}$ million instructions in one second. An alarm system operates if a patient's condition becomes critical.

Signals fed into a computer are either in digital or analog form. The latter is one which uses a variable voltage or current of electricity to convey a variable signal. For example, if body temperature is being measured then 36.8°C might be represented by 1 volt. A change of temperature in either direction could be represented by an increase or decrease of 1 millivolt for each 0.1°C.

Digital computers can undertake work of much greater complexity, compared with analog computers. Because of this the output from analog computers is often converted, at a rate of about 50 000 signals a second, into digital signals. The output from the digital computer is fed into devices such as television monitors and to magnetic tape for record purposes. A digital system uses a number of on/off states to represent a binary number that is proportional to the measurement being made.

THE BINARY OR TWO SYSTEM

All the work done in this book, so far, has been based on the 'tens' or denary number system. Many other number systems can be used, but for the purpose of computer work the binary or 'two' system is all important. In the binary system the symbols 2, 3, 4, 5, 6, 7, 8 and 9 are not used. All numbers are represented by just two digits, 1 and 0.

Conversion from the denary to the binary system

All binary numbers are expressed as a value of two, that is a power of two. To convert a number all that is necessary is to repeatedly divide by two until there is no remainder. At each stage of the division process the number is either equally divided or there is a remainder of one. The binary number is obtained from the collection of remainders, 0 is written when the number is exactly divided.

Examples

Convert the denary number 251 into a binary number:

	Remainder = binary number	*Remainder (as a power of two)*
$251 \div 2 = 125$	1	(2^0)
$125 \div 2 = 62$	1	(2^1)

$62 \div 2 =$	31	0	(2^2)
$31 \div 2 =$	15	1	(2^3)
$15 \div 2 =$	7	1	(2^4)
$7 \div 2 =$	3	1	(2^5)
$3 \div 2 =$	1	1	(2^6)
$1 \div 2 =$	0	1	(2^7)

Thus we have as a series of remainders the digits 11111011. These digits represent the binary number and in this form can be recognized by a digital computer as easily as we recognize 251. In the computer circuits 1 might be shown by switching to the 'on' position whereas 0 would be the 'off' position. Note that the digits are written horizontally so that 2^0 is on the right and is preceded by 2^1; 2^2 and so on, in the same way that units, tens and hundreds are written in the denary system.

Next, convert the denary number 39 into a binary number:

		Remainder
$39 \div 2 =$	19	1
$19 \div 2 =$	9	1
$9 \div 2 =$	4	1
$4 \div 2 =$	2	0
$2 \div 2 =$	1	0
$1 \div 2 =$	0	1

Therefore the denary number 39 = the binary number 100111.

Conversion to the denary system from the binary system

The binary number is a row of digits that indicates the powers of two in a progressive manner, starting from the digit on the right. Thus the binary number 111110011 is considered in the following order:

Binary number		*Denary equivalent*
1	$\times 2^0 =$	1
1	$\times 2^1 =$	2
0	$\times 2^2 =$	0
1	$\times 2^3 =$	8
1	$\times 2^4 =$	16
1	$\times 2^5 =$	32
1	$\times 2^6 =$	64
1	$\times 2^7 =$	128
$\therefore$11111011	=	251

Addition

Computers can easily add and subtract by using binary numbers, although the rules appear to be slightly different. The rules to remember are:

1st	$0 + 0 = 0$
2nd	$1 + 0 = 1$
3rd	$1 + 1 = 10$

Care must be taken not to confuse 10 in the third rule with ten in the denary system. As we can only count up to two, $1 + 1 = 0$ with 1 carried over to the next position. The principle is the same that is used when we add nine and one in the denary system; the sum is ten so we place 0 in the units position and carry 1 over to the tens position.

Example

Denary number		*Binary number*
50	=	110010
+44	=	+101100
94	=	1011110

To check the answer we can convert 1011110 back to the denary system:

$$\begin{aligned}
0 \times 2^0 &= 0 \\
1 \times 2^1 &= 2 \\
1 \times 2^2 &= 4 \\
1 \times 2^3 &= 8 \\
1 \times 2^4 &= 16 \\
0 \times 2^5 &= 0 \\
1 \times 2^6 &= \underline{64} \\
& \quad 94
\end{aligned}$$

Therefore the denary number 94 = the binary number 1011110.

Subtraction

The rules for subtraction are:

1st	$1 - 1 = 0$
2nd	$10 - 1 = 1$
3rd	$1 - 0 = 1$

When looking at the second rule it must be remembered that the digit on the left is twice the value of the digit to the right. As the (2^0) column is empty, as indicated by the nought, a digit is borrowed from the next highest column (2^1), therefore $10 - 1 = 1$. If this is still not clear think in terms of powers of 2, e.g.

$$\underbrace{2^1 - 2^0}_{\text{binary}} = \underbrace{2 - 1 = 1}_{\text{denary}}$$

Example

Denary number	*Binary number*	
54	110110	
–49	–110001	
5	000101	= 101 as the noughts on the left can be ignored

Once again we can check the answer by converting back to the denary system:

$$\begin{aligned} 1 \times 2^0 &= 1 \\ 0 \times 2^1 &= 0 \\ 1 \times 2^2 &= \underline{4} \\ &\ 5 \end{aligned}$$

The binary system is not difficult once the principles have been grasped. Computers certainly operate at a tremendous speed using binary numbers. When calculations have been completed the output from the computer may take the form of 'hard copy' from a teleprinter or lineprinter, a view of the answer on a television screen, or the answers may be produced on punched cards, paper tape or magnetic tape.

Exercises

1. Convert the following denary numbers to the binary scale:
(*a*) 54 (*b*) 47 (*c*) 23 (*d*) 35 (*e*) 143

2. Convert these binary numbers to the denary scale:
(*a*) 11011 (*b*) 10001 (*c*) 11010 (*d*) 110 (*e*) 101010101

3. Add the following numbers and express the answers in the denary scale.
(*a*) 110011 + 101110 + 110001
(*b*) 101 + 1011 + 10000
(*c*) 1001 + 1101 + 100110

4. Subtract the following and express the answers in the denary scale.
(*a*) 100101 – 10101
(*b*) 110110 – 101000
(*c*) 110011 – 11101

Appendix: Useful Tables

METRIC WEIGHTS

1000 micrograms	= 1 milligram
10 milligrams	= 1 centigram
10 centigrams	= 1 decigram
10 decigrams	= 1 gram
10 grams	= 1 decagram
10 decagrams	= 1 hectogram
10 hectograms	= 1 kilogram
1000 kilograms	= 1 tonne

METRIC CAPACITY

10 centimils	= 1 decimil
10 decimils	= 1 mil (1 millilitre)
10 millilitres	= 1 centilitre
10 centilitres	= 1 decilitre
10 decilitres	= 1 litre
10 litres	= 1 decalitre
10 decalitres	= 1 hectolitre

BASIC S.I. UNITS

Physical quantity	*Name of unit*	*Symbol*
Mass	kilogram	kg
Length	metre	m
Time	second	s
Electric current	Ampere	A
Temperature	degree kelvin	K
Luminous intensity	candela	cd
Amount of substance	mole	mol

Prefixes used for multiples

Figure	*Prefix*	*Sign*
10^{-12}	pico	p
10^{-9}	nano	n
10^{-6}	micro	μ
10^{-3}	milli	m
10^{3}	kilo	k
10^{6}	mega	M
10^{9}	giga	G
10^{12}	tera	T

DEFINITIONS

A dietetic Calorie is the amount of heat required to raise the temperature of 1 litre (1000 cm^3) of water 1°C and is equal to 4.184 kilojoules.

A British Thermal Unit is the amount of heat required to raise the temperature of 1 pound of water 1°F.

1 Therm equals 100 000 British Thermal Units.

1 British Thermal Unit equals $\frac{1}{4}$ dietetic Calorie.

1 Therm equals 25 200 dietetic Calories.

CALORIE VALUE OF FOODSTUFFS

1 gram of fat will produce 9 Calories or 38 kilojoules.
1 gram of protein will produce 4 Calories or 17 kilojoules.
1 gram of carbohydrate will produce 4 Calories or 17 kilojoules.

WEIGHTS AND HEIGHTS

Average Weight and Height of Children and Young People

Boys			*Girls*	
Weight (kg)	*Height (cm)*	*Age*	*Weight (kg)*	*Height (cm)*
3.4	50.6	Birth	3.36	50.2
10.07	75.2	1 year	9.75	74.2
12.56	87.5	2 years	12.29	86.6
14.61	96.2	3 years	14.42	95.7
16.51	103.4	4 years	16.42	103.2
18.89	110.0	5 years	18.58	109.4
21.91	117.5	6 years	21.09	115.9
24.54	124.1	7 years	23.68	122.3
27.26	130.0	8 years	26.35	128.0
29.94	135.5	9 years	28.94	132.9
32.61	140.3	10 years	31.89	138.6
35.2	144.2	11 years	35.74	144.7
38.28	146.6	12 years	39.74	151.9
42.18	155.0	13 years	44.95	157.1
48.81	162.7	14 years	49.17	159.6
54.48	167.8	15 years	51.48	161.1
58.83	171.6	16 years	53.07	162.2
61.78	172.7	17 years	54.02	162.5
63.05	174.5	18 years	54.39	162.5

Average Weight of Adults aged 30

Height (cm)	*Weight (kg)*		
	Small build	*Medium build*	*Large build*
Women			
152.5	48.5	53.9	60.7
157.5	51.2	56.6	63.9
162.5	53.9	59.8	67.5
167.5	57.1	63.4	71.6
172.5	60.2	67.0	75.7
178.0	63.4	70.2	78.9
Men			
167.5	58.4	64.8	72.9
172.5	61.6	68.4	77.0
177.5	65.7	72.9	82.0
183	70.7	78.4	87.9
188	75.7	83.8	94.2

DOMESTIC EQUIVALENTS (APPROXIMATE)

1 teaspoon	=	5 ml
1 dessertspoon	=	10 ml
1 tablespoon	=	20 ml
1 sherryglass	=	60 ml
1 teacup	=	142 ml
1 breakfastcup	=	230 ml
1 tumbler	=	285 ml

NORMAL VALUES

	S.I. units	*Old units*
Blood		
Bleeding time	1–6 minutes	1–6 minutes
Clotting time	4–10 minutes	4–10 minutes
Haemoglobin	12–18 g/dl	12–18 mg/100 ml
pH	7.35–7.45	7.35–7.45
pCO_2	5–6 kPa	38–45 mmHg
pO_2	11–15 kPa	80–110 mmHg
Platelets	150–400 × 10^9/litre	150 000–400 000 mm^3
Red cells	4–6 × 10^{12}/litre	4 million–6 million/mm
White cells	4–11 × 10^9/litre	4000–11 000/mm^3
Plasma		
Bicarbonate	21–28 mmol/litre	21–28 mEq/litre
Chloride	98–107 mmol/litre	98–107 mEq/litre
Glucose (fasting)	2.5–4.7 mmol/litre	45–80 mg/100 ml
Potassium	3.6–5.0 mmol/litre	3.5–5.0 mEq/litre
Sodium	135–145 mmol/litre	135–145 mEq/litre
Urea	3–7 mmol/litre	20–40 mg/100 ml
Urine		
Creatinine	10.0–15.0 mmol/litre	1.1–1.7 g/24 hours
Urea	170–580 mmol/litre	1.0–3.5 g/100 ml
S.G.	1002–1040	1002–1040
CSF		
Glucose	2.8–3.9 mmol/litre	45–70 mg/100 ml
Protein	150–300 mg/litre	15–30 mg/100 ml

Answers to Questions

Chapter 2

page 9

(*1*) 80 (*2*) 16 (*3*) 21 (*4*) 45 (*5*) 39 (*6*) 18 (*7*) 6

page 13

(*1*) *b, d, f* (*2*) *b, c, e* (*3*) *a, b, d* (*4*) (*a*) $2 \times 2 \times 3$ (*b*) 2×7 (*c*) 5×7 (*d*) 2×19 (*e*) $2 \times 3 \times 23$ (*f*) $2 \times 2 \times 5 \times 19$ (*g*) $2 \times 2 \times 3 \times 7 \times 11$ (*h*) $3 \times 5 \times 5 \times 7$

Chapter 3

page 18

(*1*) $\frac{9}{16}$ (*2*) $\frac{2}{3}$ (*3*) $\frac{3}{7}$ (*4*) $\frac{10}{11}$ (*5*) — (*6*) $\frac{1}{16}$ (*7*) $\frac{3}{16}$ (*8*) $\frac{5}{16}$ (*9*) $\frac{5}{8}$ (*10*) $\frac{1}{2}$ (*11*) $\frac{1}{4}$ (*12*) $\frac{1}{20}$ (*13*) $\frac{1}{4}$ (*14*) $\frac{3}{10}$ (*15*) $\frac{3}{4}$ (*16*) $\frac{4}{5}$ (*17*) $\frac{3}{5}$ (*18*) $\frac{7}{20}$ (*19*) $\frac{1}{5}$ (*20*) $\frac{1}{2}$ (*21*) $\frac{3}{20}$ (*22*) $\frac{3}{4}$ (*23*) 40p (*24*) 50p (*25*) £1.75 (*26*) 25p (*27*) £1.25 (*28*) 40 seconds (*29*) 55 seconds (*30*) 20 cm (*31*) 70 cm (*32*) 500 m (*33*) 750 m

page 21

(*1*) $\frac{5}{10}, \frac{7}{14}, \frac{11}{22}, \frac{20}{40}$ (*2*) $\frac{6}{8}, \frac{12}{16}, \frac{6}{8}, \frac{9}{12}$ (*3*) $\frac{6}{10}, \frac{15}{25}, \frac{21}{35}, \frac{36}{60}$ (*4*) $\frac{1}{3}$ (*5*) $\frac{1}{5}$ (*6*) $\frac{1}{3}$ (*7*) $\frac{3}{4}$ (*8*) $\frac{5}{16}$ (*9*) $\frac{1}{4}$ (*10*) $\frac{1}{2}$ (*11*) $\frac{1}{4}$ (*12*) $\frac{1}{4}$ (*13*) $\frac{1}{8}$ (*14*) $\frac{1}{100}$ (*15*) $\frac{1}{50}$ (*16*) $\frac{1}{100}$ (*17*) $\frac{1}{2}$ (*18*) $\frac{3}{4}$ (*19*) $\frac{1}{20}$ (*20*) $\frac{2}{3}$

page 23

(*1*) $2\frac{1}{2}$ (*2*) $1\frac{1}{4}$ (*3*) $2\frac{1}{3}$ (*4*) $1\frac{3}{5}$ (*5*) $2\frac{3}{4}$ (*6*) 6 (*7*) $2\frac{7}{11}$ (*8*) $2\frac{4}{7}$ (*9*) $2\frac{1}{3}$ (*10*) $3\frac{5}{9}$

page 24

(*1*) $\frac{4}{3}$ (*2*) $\frac{5}{3}$ (*3*) $\frac{11}{4}$ (*4*) $\frac{25}{8}$ (*5*) $\frac{35}{8}$ (*6*) $\frac{57}{8}$ (*7*) $\frac{37}{10}$ (*8*) $\frac{43}{10}$ (*9*) $\frac{65}{7}$ (*10*) $\frac{517}{100}$

page 27

(*1*) $\frac{8}{9}$ (2) $\frac{3}{4}$ (*3*) $\frac{2}{3}$ (*4*) $\frac{1}{2}$ (*5*) $\frac{7}{10}$ (*6*) $\frac{17}{20}$ (*7*) $\frac{1}{12}$ (*8*) $1\frac{1}{18}$ (*9*) $\frac{5}{7}$ (*10*) $\frac{9}{16}$ (*11*) $1\frac{2}{5}$ (*12*) $\frac{3}{8}$ (*13*) $\frac{1}{4}$ (*14*) $1\frac{1}{10}$ (*15*) $\frac{34}{75}$

page 30

(*1*) $\frac{1}{8}$ (2) $\frac{3}{16}$ (*3*) $\frac{1}{4}$ (*4*) $1\frac{3}{4}$ (*5*) $1\frac{1}{3}$ (*6*) $\frac{1}{6}$ (*7*) 1 (*8*) $\frac{4}{15}$ (*9*) $1\frac{5}{7}$ (*10*) $\frac{1}{2}$ litre

page 32

(*1*) $\frac{6}{7}$ (2) $2\frac{2}{9}$ (*3*) $2\frac{1}{2}$ (*4*) $3\frac{1}{2}$ (*5*) $\frac{5}{7}$ (*6*) 3 (*7*) 4 (*8*) $3\frac{3}{4}$ (*9*) $\frac{6}{35}$ (*10*) $\frac{3}{22}$ (*11*) 6 (*12*) $\frac{2}{3}$ (*13*) 2 (*14*) $\frac{1}{4}$ (*15*) 20 (*16*) $5\frac{3}{5}$ (*17*) 8 (*18*) $102\frac{2}{3}$ (*19*) $2\frac{4}{9}$ (*20*) $3\frac{3}{4}$

page 34

(*1*) $1\frac{1}{9}$ (2) $\frac{9}{14}$ (*3*) $5\frac{1}{2}$ (*4*) $11\frac{2}{3}$ (*5*) $\frac{3}{4}$ (*6*) $\frac{7}{24}$ (*7*) $\frac{19}{22}$ (*8*) $\frac{2}{3}$ (*9*) $\frac{8}{9}$ (*10*) $1\frac{1}{3}$ (*11*) 14 (*12*) $\frac{4}{5}$ (*13*) 30 (*14*) 14 rolls; 15p left over; 3 decorations (*15*) £204

Chapter 4

page 38

(*1*) $5\frac{1}{5}$ (2) $2\frac{1}{2}$ (*3*) $3\frac{1}{4}$ (*4*) $\frac{3}{5}$ (*5*) $\frac{3}{50}$ (*6*) $\frac{3}{500}$ (*7*) $4\frac{1}{8}$ (*8*) $2\frac{11}{20}$ (*9*) $1\frac{1}{20}$ (*10*) $\frac{1}{2000}$

page 39

(*1*) 0.35 (2) 0.12 (*3*) 0.3125 (*4*) 0.825 (*5*) 0.28125 (*6*) 0.6625 (*7*) 2.65 (*8*) 3.46875 (*9*) 2.825 (*10*) 3.456

page 43

(*1*) (*a*) 7 (*b*) 17 (*c*) 0.07 (*d*) 30.4 (*e*) 73.2 (2) (*a*) 320 (*b*) 1704 (*c*) 0.7 (*d*) 100.7 (*e*) 1310 (*3*) 1.449 (*4*) 18.7 (*5*) 96.52 (*6*) 0.584 (*7*) 2.1994 (*8*) 0.913 (*9*) 0.0913 (*10*) 0.0913 (*11*) 0.00231 (*12*) 27.4104 (*13*) 2.050642 (*14*) 0.421875 (*15*) 65.596 (*16*) 93.5415

page 45
(*1*) (*a*) 0.9 (*b*) 0.4 (*c*) 4 (*d*) 0.011 (*e*) 300 (*f*) 0.056 (*g*) 3.309 (*h*) 0.04 (*i*) 42.1 (*j*) 50 (*2*) (*a*) 99; 990; 9900 (*b*) 87.9; 879; 8790 (*c*) 6; 60; 600 (*d*) 0.1; 1; 10 (*e*) 6.5; 65; 650 (*f*) 4.08; 40.8; 408 (*g*) 932.8; 9328; 93 280 (*h*) 70.5; 705; 7050 (*i*) 400.2; 4002; 40 020 (*3*) (*a*) 75; 7.5; 0.75 (*b*) 6.232; 0.6232; 0.06232 (*c*) 0.423; 0.0423; 0.00423 (*d*) 0.0025; 0.00025; 0.000025 (*4*) (*a*) 7.2 (*b*) 0.93 (*c*) 0.012 (*d*) 70.08 (*5*) (*a*) $\frac{9}{10}$ (*b*) $\frac{9}{100}$ (*c*) $\frac{1}{4}$ (*d*) $2\frac{1}{4}$ (*e*) $\frac{56}{125}$ (*f*) $2\frac{19}{250}$ (*g*) $\frac{1}{400}$ (*6*) (*a*) 0.0575 (*b*) 0.00648 (*c*) 157.2 (*d*) 49.602 (*e*) 90.712 (*f*) 262.2048 (*7*) (*a*) 0.3 (*b*) 0.83 (*c*) 0.1 (*d*) 0.27 (*e*) 0.142857 (*8*) (*a*) 24 800 (*b*) 276 000 (*c*) 976 000 (*d*) 0.0076 (*e*) 0.88 (*f*) 0.094 (*g*) 0.067

Chapter 5

page 52
(*1*) 1000 mg (*2*) 1000 ml (*3*) 3.155 m (*4*) 0.25 litre (*5*) 1.5 g (*6*) 1750 ml (*7*) 0.05 litre (*8*) 1080 ml (*9*) 62 mg (*10*) 0.96 litre (*11*) 0.0459 litre (*12*) 9600 g (*13*) 40.364 litres (*14*) 1.272 g (*15*) 7 litres, 531 ml (*16*) 23.54 mg, 0.02354 g (*17*) 750 μg (*18*) 0.75 mm

pages 57–60
(*1*) (*a*) 0.225 kg; 0.495 lb (*b*) 3.55 kg; 7.81 lb (*c*) 0.221 kg; 0.4862 lb (*d*) 1.4 kg; 3.08 lb (*2*) (*a*) 0.227 kg; 227 g (*b*) 4.545 kg; 4545 g (*c*) 1 kg; 1000 g (*d*) 2.5 kg; 2500 g (*3*) (*a*) 6 st 4 lb; 7 st $7\frac{3}{5}$ lb; 8 st $11\frac{1}{5}$ lb; 9 st $1\frac{3}{5}$ lb; 9 st $10\frac{2}{5}$ lb; 15 st 10 lb (*b*) $60\frac{2}{3}$ kg; 4 st $7\frac{1}{2}$ lb (*4*) (*a*) 150 ml; 0.15 litre (*b*) 315 ml; 0.315 litre (*c*) 280 ml; 0.28 litre (*5*) (*a*) $1\frac{2}{5}$ fl oz; $3\frac{1}{2}$ fl oz; $52\frac{1}{2}$ fl oz; $17\frac{1}{2}$ fl oz; $13\frac{1}{8}$ fl oz (*b*) 0.57 litre; 0.057 litre; 14.3 ml (*6*) 1.2 g (*7*) 0.8 g; 1086 mg; 1 lb; 0.75 kg (*8*) 300 cm^3; 0.75 pint; 0.5 litre; 625 ml; 180 fl oz (*9*) 0.225 litre; 2.25 decilitres; 2.25 millilitres (*10*) 23 trays (*11*) £20.274 (*12*) 350 g carbohydrate; 125 g protein; 25 g fat

page 62

(*1*) (*a*) 37.84 in (*b*) 1.32 in (*c*) 5.12 in (*d*) 1.48 in (*e*) 3.4 in (*f*) 50.52 in (*g*) 0.84 in (*h*) 0.56 in (*i*) 0.71 in (*2*) (*a*) 1050 mm (*b*) 2200 mm (*c*) 43.75 mm (*d*) 562.5 mm (*e*) 950 mm (*f*) 72.5 mm (*g*) 365 mm (*h*) 1420 mm (*i*) 1800 mm (*3*) 90; 55; 87.4 cm (*4*) (*a*) 143 lb (*b*) 290.4 lb (*c*) 105.6 lb (*d*) 46.2 lb (*e*) 233.2 lb (*f*) 72.6 lb (*g*) 167.2 lb (*h*) 35.2 lb (*i*) 114.4 lb (*5*) (*a*) 33.6 kg (*b*) 69.5 kg (*c*) 15 kg (*d*) 41.8 kg (*e*) 29.0 kg (*f*) 17.7 kg (*g*) 30 kg (*h*) 30.9 kg (*i*) 9.55 kg (*6*) (*a*) 50 kg (*b*) 51.7 kg (*c*) 66.3 kg (*d*) 89 kg (*e*) 82.7 kg (*f*) 95.4 kg (*7*) 8.1 kg (*8*) 283.6 mg (*9*) (*a*) 18.6 oz (*b*) 7.7 oz (*c*) 66.85 oz (*d*) 29.1 oz (*e*) 22.4 oz (*f*) 11.2 oz (*g*) 26.3 oz (*h*) 19.3 oz (*i*) 16.5 oz (*10*) (*a*) 1511 ml (*b*) 798 ml (*c*) 941 ml (*d*) 131 ml (*e*) 428 ml (*f*) 117 ml (*g*) 912 ml (*h*) 274 ml (*i*) 2366 ml

Chapter 6

page 69

(*1*) (*a*) $\frac{1}{100}$; 0.01 (*b*) $\frac{1}{10}$; 0.1 (*c*) $\frac{3}{20}$; 0.15 (*d*) $\frac{1}{5}$; 0.2 (*e*) $\frac{2}{5}$; 0.4 (*f*) $\frac{1}{2}$; 0.5 (*g*) $\frac{3}{4}$; 0.75 (*h*) $\frac{9}{10}$; 0.9 (2) (*a*) 1% (*b*) 5% (*c*) 24% (*d*) 35% (*e*) 9% (*f*) 96% (*g*) 75% (*h*) $87\frac{1}{2}$% (*3*) (*a*) 30% (*b*) 75% (*c*) 42% (*d*) 1% (*e*) 66% (*f*) 25% (*g*) $30\frac{1}{2}$% (*h*) 39.3% (*4*) 8 nurses (*5*) 120 ml (*6*) 200 ml (*7*) $66\frac{2}{3}$% (*8*) £21.13 (*9*) 340 adults (*10*) £660 per annum

Chapter 10

pages 108–110

(*1*) (*a*) 0.8 ml (*b*) 0.8 ml (*c*) 0.6 ml (*d*) 0.75 ml (*e*) 0.3 ml (*f*) 1.1 ml (*g*) 0.75 ml (2) (*a*) 1 in 40 (*b*) 1 in 5000 (*c*) 1 in 150 (*d*) 1 in 200 (*e*) 1 in 200 (*f*) 1 in 250 (*3*) (*a*) 1.25% (*b*) 0.1% (*c*) 2.5% (*d*) 1% (*4*) (*a*) 1:40 (*b*) 1:33 (*c*) 1:25 (*d*) 1:100 (*e*) 1:20 (*5*) (*a*) 2 ml; 1 in 50 (*b*) 402; 10% (*c*) 300 ml; 1 in 100 (*d*) 1200 ml;

$1\frac{1}{4}$% (*e*) 640 ml; 1 in 160 (*f*) 250 ml; 0.1% (*g*) 3 ml; 1 in 10000 (*h*) 8 ml; 1 in 5 (*i*) 3 ml; 1 in 40 (*j*) 10 ml; 1 in 200 (*k*) $\frac{1}{2}$ oz; $1\frac{2}{3}$% (*l*) 1 ml; 1 in 500 (*m*) 320 ml; 1 in 80 (*n*) 40 ml; $1\frac{1}{4}$%

Chapter 11

page 116
(*1*) 2.5 ml (*2*) $\frac{1}{4}$ tablet (*3*) 5 ml (*4*) 10 ml (*5*) 0.2 ml (*6*) 0.6 ml (*7*) 1.6 ml (*8*) 8 ml

pages 116–117
(*1*) Draw up $\frac{3}{4}$ of the Omnopon and discard the remainder (*2*) 3600 ml (*3*) 625 ml (*4*) 400 ml; 800 ml (*5*) $\frac{5}{8}$ (0.625) ml (*6*) $1\frac{1}{3}$ ml (*7*) Pethidine 75 mg; promethazine 37.5 mg (*8*) 125 ml (*9*) Take 400 ml of 1 in 1000, add 200 ml water (*10*) 75 ml (*11*) 80 ml (*12*) $1\frac{1}{3}$ ml (*13*) 900 ml (*14*) 20 ml (*15*) 4 litres; 750 ml (*16*) 125 ml (*17*) 125 ml

Chapter 12

page 128
(*3*) (*a*) 37.4°F (*b*) 64.4°F (*c*) 77.9°F (*d*) 212°F (*e*) 96.8°F (*f*) 107.6°F (*g*) 122°F (*h*) 158°F (*4*) (*a*) 5°C (*b*) 25°C (*c*) 13°C (*d*) 40°C (*e*) 30°C (*f*) 26°C (*g*) 185.5°C (*h*) 100°C (*5*) (*a*) false (*b*) true (*c*) true (*d*) false (*e*) false (*f*) false (*g*) false

Chapter 13

page 142
(*1*) $2\frac{1}{4}$ hours (*2*) 6 hours 21 minutes

page 148
(*1*) (*a*) 3.3 kg (*b*) 4.6 kg (*c*) 5.2 kg (*2*) (*a*) 750 to 1000 ml and 2100 to 2700 kJ (500 to 650 Calories) (*b*) 600 to 800 ml; 1680 to 2160 kJ (400 to 520 Calories) (*3*) 840 to 1120 ml; 2352 to 3024 kJ (560 to 728 Calories)

Chapter 15

page 173

(*1*) 140°F; 41°F; 68°F; 95°F; 151°F; 154°F; 167°F; 198°F
(2) 10°C; 7°C; 22°C; $35\frac{1}{2}$°C; 42°C; 53°C; 59°C; 93°C; 37°C

page 174

(*1*) No (*2*) 4.45 kg (*3*) $4\frac{1}{2}$ weeks (*4*) No (*5*) Yes

page 161

(*5*) (*a*) 99.4°F = 37.4°C (*b*) 102.6°F = 39.2°C (*c*) 95
(*d*) 11.5°F = 38.1°C

Chapter 17

page 186

(*1*) (*a*) 54 = 110110 (*b*) 47 = 101111 (*c*) 23 = 10111
(*d*) 35 = 100011 (*e*) 143 = 10001111 (2) (*a*) 27 (*b*) 17
(*c*) 53 (*d*) 6 (*e*) 341 (*3*) (*a*) 10010010 = 146
(b) 100000 = 32 (*c*) 111100 = 60 (*4*) (*a*) 10000 = 16
(*b*) 1110 = 14 (*c*) 10110 = 22

Index